70 Of The E
Barbecu

That Will Allow You To Cook Up A Great Feast In The Summer

Samantha Michaels

Table of Contents

ENJOY YOUR FREE DOWNLOADS? PLEASE CLICK HERE TO GIVE ME SOME REVIEWS ON THE BOOK ...APPRECIATE IT!!

Introduction

Most people these days will cook only meat on their barbecues, but cooking fish on them is wonderful as well. Actually cooking fish on a barbecue on a barbecue isn't that difficult and you may be surprised at how easy it is to achieve the kinds of results that more experienced chefs achieved when cooking in this way.

Certainly when it comes to cooking fish on a barbecue you can use either a solid fuel (charcoal) or gas fired one to do so. Plus it is also important that you actually have the right equipment at hand when you do start cooking and allow yourself plenty of time to prepare the fish.

The kind of equipment needed for cooking fish on a barbecue includes the following:

1. A fish basket

2. Some form of lining for the fish, such as aluminum foil or things like banana leaves or corn husks which can be wrapped around the fish being cooked.

3. If you are intending to bake the fish rather than grill it then of course use a barbecue fitted with a hood.

4. You can of course also smoke fish on your barbecue if you want but in order to do this you will need to invest money in a good smoker box plus the wood chips.

Another important thing to consider when cooking such food on a barbecue is that you use only the finest quality fish you can. The things to look for when choosing your fish are as follows:

1. That the fish you choose has a nice sea smell to it. This will clearly indicate the fish you have brought is fresh.

2. Look closely at the eyes of the fish if they are sunken rather than looking bright don't cook them. The fish isn't at all fresh and could lead to health issues after it has been eaten.

3. Finally don't be afraid to touch the fish and push down on it. If the flesh of the fish is firm and springs back after it has been touched then you know what you are eating is still good.

As for cooking the fish it is important that you prepare the barbecue before you do. Below are the things that should be done before you begin cooking fish on your barbecue.

1. If you are going to be using a fish basket for cooking your fish on the barbecue then line it first with aluminum foil. This will not only help to cook through evenly but will help it to retain moisture. Also if you are going to line the fish basket with foil make sure that the shiny side is facing towards the fish.

2. If you haven't marinated the fish first before you place it on the barbecue it is a good ide to oil and season it first to taste.

3. If you would like the fish to retain as much moisture as possible then it is best to remove the scales first.

4. Make sure that you preheat the barbecue before you begin cooking. Follow the barbecue manufacturer's instructions about preparing it for cooking.

5. Finally decide whether you will cook the fish on the plate or grill. If you intend to cook

the fish on a plate in a basket then make sure that you don't allow it to come in to direct contact with it.

In this particular recipe book are a variety of wonderful array of amazing fresh fish and shell fish dishes that you may want to try out on your barbecue this summer or next.

Chapter 1 – Fish Barbecue Recipes

Recipe 1 – Fresh Citrus Salmon

This particular recipe comes with quite a tangy taste, which helps to enhance the flavor of the salmon further.

Ingredients

4 Salmon Fillets With Skin Left On
2 Small Lemons
2 Medium Oranges
1 Large Lime

100ml Freshly Squeezed Lemon Juice
100ml Freshly Squeezed Orange Juice
2 Large Garlic Cloves Divided
Freshly Ground Black Pepper
Sea Salt
50ml Freshly Squeezed Lime Juice
Olive Oil
4 Tablespoons Balsamic Vinegar
2 Teaspoons Freshly Chopped Dill

Instructions

1. Wash the salmon fillets thoroughly before then patting dry and drizzling them with some olive oil and sprinkling over them some sea salt and pepper on the skin side and rub it in. Then place in the refrigerator for 30 minutes.

2. Cut the lemon, lime and oranges into segments making sure that you retain as much of their juices as possible. Then mix these segments with some olive oil and ½ crushed garlic clove. Now place in the refrigerator.

3. Next you need to combine the freshly cut dill with 1 garlic clove that has been crushed, the lime, lemon and orange juice and a little olive oil, salt and pepper. Once you have done

this you remove the salmon fillets from the refrigerator and place them in a shallow dish and pour over this marinade. Cover the dish and replace in the refrigerator and leave the salmon to marinate in the dill for at least 2 hours.

4. Once two hours is up remove the salmon fillets from the refrigerator and as the barbecue warms up this will allow them to come up to room temperature. Allow the salmon to be out of the refrigerator for 20 minutes before you then place on the barbecue.

5. Before you place the salmon on the barbecue rub the grate with a clove of garlic and then place the fish on it skin side down. After two minutes you must turn the salmon over and allow it to cook for a further two minutes. Also it is important to place some sort of cover over the salmon such as saucepan lid that is well ventilated. Once cooked let the salmon fillets rest for 3 minutes before serving. When you serve the salmon place on the plate a small salad made up of lettuce, cherry tomatoes and drizzle some balsamic vinegar around the plate.

Recipe 2 – Marinated Barbecued Swordfish

The use of white wine, soy sauce, garlic and lemon juice help to bring out more of the swordfishes amazing flavor as well as help to cook it better on the barbecue.

Ingredients

4 Swordfish Steaks
4 Garlic Cloves
75ml White Wine
4 Tablespoons Lemon Juice
2 Tablespoons Soy Sauce
2 Tablespoons Olive Oil
1 Tablespoon Savory Seasoning
¼ Teaspoon Salt
1/8 Teaspoon Freshly Ground Black Pepper

Instructions

1. In a shallow dish you whisk together the garlic, white wine, soy sauce, lemon juice, olive oil, salt and pepper and savory seasoning. Now place the swordfish steaks into the dish and turn them over so that they are coated in the marinade you have just made fully. Then place in the refrigerator for one

hour making sure that turn the steaks over frequently during this time.

2. After one hour remove the steaks from the refrigerator and turn on the barbecue. Whilst the barbecue is heating up this will provide the steaks with sufficient time to reach room temperature and so will help to ensure that they then cook properly.

3. As soon as the barbecue has heated up it needs to be as hot as possible you lightly oil the grate and then place the swordfish steaks on to it. Cook for 5 to 6 minutes on each side before then removing to a clean plate and garnish them with some freshly chopped parsley and wedges of lemon.

Recipe 3 – Grilled Sea Bass With Garlic Sauce

If you have never cooked sea bass on a barbecue before this is a very simple and easy recipe that you may want to try. You will find that the garlic butter actually complements the mild flavors of what is a very light and flaky fish.

Ingredients

907grams Sea Bass
3 Tablespoons Butter
1 ½ Tablespoons Extra Virgin Olive Oil
1 Tablespoon Freshly Finely Chopped Italian Parsley
2 Garlic Cloves Minced
¼ Teaspoon Garlic Powder
¼ Teaspoon Paprika
¼ Teaspoon Onion Powder
Lemon Pepper And Salt To Taste

Instructions

1. In a bowl combine together the garlic powder, onion powder, paprika, lemon pepper and salt and then sprinkle this over both sides

of the sea bass. Then place in the refrigerator to rest whilst you go ahead and prepare the garlic sauce.

2.   To make the garlic sauce into a small saucepan place the butter minced garlic cloves and parsley and heat on a low heat until all the butter has melted. Then place to one side ready to use later on.

3.   When it comes to cooking the sea bass on the barbecue you need to do so on a medium high heat and ensure that the grate has been oiled first. Now place the sea bass on the barbecue and cook it for 7 minutes before then turning it over. After you have turned the fish over brush some of the garlic sauce over the top and then allow the sea bass to cook for a further 7 minutes.

4.   As soon as the necessary cooking time has elapsed the fish should flake easily and this is the right time to remove from the heat. Place the fish on a clean plate and then drizzle over some olive oil and some more of the garlic sauce.

Recipe 4 – Barbecued Salmon With Soy & Brown Sugar Marinade

The mixture of brown sugar, soy sauce, lemon and garlic provides the perfect sweet and salty taste to the rich flavor of the salmon.

Ingredients

700grams Salmon Fillet
1 Tablespoon Lemon Zest
1 Tablespoon Minced Garlic Clove
5 Tablespoons Soy Sauce
4 Tablespoons Dark Brown Soft Sugar
5 Tablespoons Water
4 Tablespoons Vegetable Oil
Freshly Ground Black Pepper To Taste

Instructions

1. In a bowl place the sugar, water, vegetable oil, lemon zest, minced garlic, pepper and soy sauce and mix together until as much of the sugar has dissolved as possible.

2. Once you have made the marinade you now place the salmon fillet into a large resealable plastic bag and pour the marinade over it.

Close the bag up and then turn it over several times to ensure that the fillet of salmon is completely covered in the marinade. Place in the refrigerator for at least 2 hours.

3. Once the two hours has passed removed the salmon from the refrigerator and start heating up the barbecue. By the time the barbecue has heated up the salmon fillet should have come up to room temperature and will be ready to start cooking.

4. To cook the salmon fillet on the barbecue you can either place it directly on to the grate that has been lightly oiled or directly on to a piece of aluminum foil that has been lightly oiled. Any marinade that remains should now be discarded.

5. You should cook each side of the salmon for between 5 and 6 minutes or when you use a fork to separate the flesh it flakes easily. Once cooked simply place on a clean plate and then allow your guests to help themselves.

Recipe 5 – Grilled Onion Butter Cod

When cooked on a barbecue you will find the cod becomes very tender and the grilled onion butter enhances not only the flavor but also the texture of this fish. Best served with some grilled potatoes and vegetables.

Ingredients

4 Cod Fillets (Each Fillet Should Weigh About 170grams)
1 Small Finely Chopped Onion
60ml White Wine
45gram Butter
1 Tablespoon Extra Virgin Olive Oil
½ Teaspoon Salt
½ Teaspoon Freshly Ground Black Pepper
1 Sliced Lemon

Instructions

1.   Whilst the barbecue is heating up you should be preparing the onion butter. To do this into a small frying pan (skillet) place the better and once it is melted to it add the finely chopped onion and allow it to cook for about 1

to 2 minutes. Then to this you add the wine and leave to simmer for 3 minutes. When this time has elapsed remove from the heat and let it cool slightly.

2.   As soon as the barbecue has reached the right temperature you should now lightly brush the cod fillets with the olive oil and sprinkle on some salt and black pepper before then placing on to the lightly oiled barbecue grill.

3.   Cook the fish on one side for about 8 minutes before then turning it over and basting with some of the butter sauce you made earlier. Now allow the fish to cook for a further 6 to 7 minutes or until you notice the flesh has begun to turn opaque. During this cooking time it is important that you baste the fish with the butter sauce a further 2 or 3 times before then removing from the heat and placing on a clean plate and serving with the wedges of lemon.

Recipe 6 – Grilled Trout With Parsley

It is best if you use a whole fish rather than fillets as you want to actually place the herbs inside the body of it. You can enjoy this particular barbecue recipe any time of the week.

Ingredients

2 x 450gram Trout (Whole Is Best)
2 Tablespoons Freshly Minced Parsley
2 Tablespoons Olive Oil
2 Tablespoons Freshly Minced Basil
1 Tablespoon Freshly Minced Rosemary
2 Freshly Minced Cloves of Garlic
½ Teaspoon Salt
½ Teaspoon Freshly Ground Black Pepper

Instructions

1. In a small bowl combine together the parsley, olive oil, basil, rosemary and garlic and then spread this evenly over the inside of the fish.

2. Now place the fish in a shallow dish, cover and place in a refrigerator for 2 hours.

3. After 2 hours have elapsed remove the trout from the refrigerator and start heating up the barbecue. Just before placing the trout on to the barbecue grill brush it with some oil and sprinkle both sides of the trout with salt and pepper.

4. Cook the trout on a medium heat for 4 to 5 minutes on each side before carefully removing it and serving the trout on a clean plate.

Recipe 7 – Barbecued Teriyaki Tuna Steaks

Fresh tuna steaks always taste best when cooked on a barbecue. If you want your teriyaki marinade to have a little bit of a kick add some paprika or freshly minced ginger to it.

Ingredients

4 Tuna Steaks (You Can Use Fillets If You Wish)
225ml Teriyaki Sauce
180ml Olive Oil
2 Garlic Cloves Minced
1 Teaspoon Freshly Ground Black Pepper

Instructions

1. Into a large resealable plastic bag pour the teriyaki sauce, olive oil, minced garlic and freshly ground black pepper. Seal the bag up and the shake vigorously to ensure that all these ingredients combine well together.

2. Now place the tuna steaks in the bag and make sure that it is tightly sealed before turning it over several times to ensure that all

the marinade coats the steaks well. Now place in the refrigerator to allow the marinade to infuse into the steaks for 30 minutes.

3.   Whilst the tuna is in the refrigerator marinating you should now heating up the barbecue. As soon as the barbecue is ready for cooking on take the tuna steaks out of the bag and place them on the oiled barbecue grill and cook until done. If there is any marinade remaining in the bag this should be discarded.

4.   As soon as the tuna steaks are cooked remove from barbecue place on clean plates and serve with a fresh crispy green salad.

Recipe 8 – Lime & Basil Tilapia

Combining lime and basil together helps to add even more flavor to the tilapia. You can either serve this barbecue fish dish with some freshly grilled vegetables or you can slice the fish and then serve it in tacos.

Ingredients

4 Tilapia Fillets (Each Weighing Around 115grams)
60ml Olive Oil
2 Tablespoons Lime Juice
Zest of 2 Limes
1 Tablespoon Freshly Minced Basil
2 Teaspoons Bourbon
1 Teaspoon Salt
Freshly Ground Pepper To Taste

Instructions

1. In a resealable plastic bag put the olive oil, lime juice and zest, freshly minced basil, bourbon, salt and pepper. Now close the bag up ensuring it is tightly sealed and shake the contents inside vigorously to make sure that they are all mixed together properly.

2. Once the marinade is prepared you now need to open the bag up and put the tilapia fillets in and seal the bag once more. After doing this turn the bag over several times to ensure that all of the fillets have been coated in the marinade and then place in a refrigerator for 30 minutes.

3. When the 30 minutes have elapsed remove the fillets from the bag and pour any marinade left in the bag into a saucepan. Whilst the barbecue is heating up you now need to heat the marinade up in the saucepan and then bring it to a low boil. As soon as the marinade starts to boil remove from the heat and place to one side.

4. Next you need to cook the Tilapia fillets. It is important that you cook this fish on a high heat and each side should be cooked for at least 3 minutes. As soon as the fish has turned opaque you should remove it from the heat and serve with some of the marinade in the saucepan drizzled over the top.

Recipe 9 – Barbecued Tuna With Honey Glaze

The lime coriander and honey help to enhance the flavor of what is quite a meaty fish further.

Ingredients

450grams Tuna Fillets
4 Tablespoons Olive Oil
4 Tablespoons Lime Juice (Fresh Would Be Best)
2 Tablespoons Balsamic Vinegar
2 Cloves Garlic Minced
1 Tablespoon Freshly Minced Ginger Root
1 Small Bunch Freshly Chopped Coriander

Honey Glaze

4 Tablespoons Honey
2 Tablespoons Olive Oil
2 Tablespoons Freshly Chopped Coriander

Instructions

1. Into a medium size bowl mix together the olive oil, lime juice, minced garlic, balsamic vinegar, freshly minced ginger root and freshly

chopped coriander. Once all these ingredients have been combined well together you add the tuna fillets and turn them over several times to ensure that each one is evenly coated in the marinade. Now cover the bowl over and place in a refrigerator and leave for several hours.

2. After several hours now is the time to start heating up the barbecue. It is important that when cooking the tuna on the barbecue you do so on a high heat. Whilst the barbecue is heating up this is the time when you should be making the honey glaze.

3. To make the honey glaze place the honey, olive oil and freshly chopped coriander in a bowl and whisk. Then set it to one side.

4. By the time you have finished making the honey glaze the barbecue should have reached the desired temperature for cooking the tuna fillets. However before you place the tuna fillets on the grill make sure that you lightly oil it first.

5. Once you have placed the tuna on the grill close the lid and allow the fillets to cook for 1 to 2 minutes before opening the lid and then turning the fillets over. Now close the lid for a

further minute then open the lid and continue to cook the tuna until it is barely done. It is important that whilst the tuna fillets are cooking you baste them regularly with the marinade.

6.   As soon as the tuna fillets are nearly cooked through you should brush both sides of them with the honey glaze and then remove from the barbecue and serve.

Recipe 10 – Blackened Fish

The great thing about cooking blackened fish on a barbecue is that you won't find your kitchen filling up with smoke.

Ingredients

6 Firm Fish Fillets
3 Tablespoons Cajun Blackening Spices
339grams Unsalted Butter Melted

Instructions

1. Heat up the barbecue until it is good and hot. Once the barbecue has reached the desired temperature now you can begin cooking the fish fillets.

2. Pour most of the melted butter into a shallow dish (leave around 12 tablespoons of the butter to one side as you will use this later when serving the fish). After pouring the melted butter into the dish dip each fillet (both sides) in it before then sprinkling some of the Cajun blackening spices over them.

3. Once this has been done place the fillets on the oiled barbecue grill and cook for about 2 minutes before then turning them over and cooking the other side for a further 2 minutes. As soon as this time has elapsed or when you feel the fillets are cooked through remove from heat and place on clean plates along with a small bowl in which some of the remaining butter has been placed that your guests can then dip the fish fillets into.

Recipe 11 – Citrus Marjoram Marinated Halibut Steak

It is important that when making the citrus marinade for this particular recipe that you use sprigs of fresh marjoram. Also it is important that you only allow the fish to marinate in the sauce for no more than 2 hours. If you marinate it for any longer than this the texture of the fish will be affected.

Ingredients

800grams Halibut Steaks
7 Tablespoons Fresh Grapefruit Juice
4 Tablespoons Olive Oil
1 Dessertspoon Freshly Chopped Marjoram
½ Teaspoon Salt
1/8 Teaspoon Freshly Ground Black Pepper

4 Springs Fresh Marjoram To Use As Garnish

Instructions

1. In a shallow dish mix together the grapefruit juice, olive oil, freshly chopped marjoram, salt and pepper.

2. To this mixture add the fish making sure you turn it over so both sides are coated in the marinade. Now cover and place in the refrigerator for 1 to 2 hours. Whilst it is marinating make sure that you turn the fish over once or twice.

3. After the marinating time has elapsed you should start heating up the barbecue, with the grill placed 4 to 6 inches above the heat source. Whilst the barbecue is heating up take the fish out of the refrigerator so that they come up to room temperature.

4. When the barbecue has heated up now place the halibut steaks into a fish basket that has been lightly oiled and place on the barbecue grill. You should cook these steaks for between 10 and 12 minutes turning them once and brushing with any marinade you have left over. Serve once the steaks have become barely opaque in the thickest part on a clean plate with the sprigs of fresh marjoram.

Recipe 12 – Grilled Red Snapper

You will need a whole red snapper for this recipe. But don't worry grilling a whole fish isn't as difficult as it sounds, especially if you have never done it before.

Ingredients

970grams Whole Red Snapper (Split and Butterflied)
60ml Achiote Paste
60ml Orange Juice
3 Tablespoons Lemon Juice
3 Tablespoons Lime Juice
(If you can use fresh orange, lemon and lime juice)

Instructions

1. In a bowl mix together the achiote paste with the orange, lemon and lime juice and spread over all surfaces of the Red Snapper. Place into a shallow dish which you then cover before putting in the refrigerator to rest for at least 2 hours.

2. Just before the fish comes out of the refrigerator start up the barbecue and place the grill about 6 inches above the heat source as you want to cook this fish on a medium heat.

3. Once the barbecue has heated up lightly oil the grill and then place the Red Snapper on it skin side down and leave it there for about 5 minutes. Then after this time turning the fish over and let it cook for a further 3 minutes. You will notice that the fish is done when the juices begin boiling and also you will find removing the central bone is easy because it simply lifts out when the fish is cooked.

4. If you would like to cook the fish in the same way that Mexican people do then try and get a banana leaf on which to place it when cooking. If you can make sure that the leaf is still wet when you place it on the grill first before adding the fish.   Not only will this prevent the fish from sticking to the grill but also help to stop it from falling apart as you turn it over.

Recipe 13 – Ginger Swordfish

An amazing marinade that really helps to bring some amazing flavors out of the swordfish.

Ingredients

6 Swordfish Steaks
175ml Teriyaki Sauce
150ml Dry Sherry
8 Garlic Cloves Freshly Minced
1 Dessertspoon Freshly Minced Ginger Root
1 Teaspoon Sesame Oil

Instructions

1. Into a saucepan (large) place the teriyaki sauce, dry sherry, garlic, ginger and sesame oil, mix and bring up to the boil. Once boiling remove the pan from the heat and set to one side to cool for 10 minutes.

2. In a shallow dish place the swordfish steaks and pour some of the marinade over the top that you made earlier. Then turn the steaks over and pour the rest of the marinade over them. Cover the dish up and place in the refrigerator for 1 ½ hours. During this time

you should make sure that you turn the Swordfish steaks over frequently.

3. About 15 minutes before you remove the fish from the refrigerator you should get the barbecue started and place the grill about 4 to 6 inches above the heat source. This type of fish should be cooked on a medium to high heat.

4. Once the barbecue has heated up you can now place the steaks on the lightly oiled grill and cook them on each side for 4 minutes. The best way of telling that the Swordfish steaks are cooked is that when prodded with a fork the meat should easily flake. Serve to your guests immediately after removing from the barbecue.

Recipe 14 – Grilled Asian Style Catfish

This is one of the simplest recipes you can use to prepare catfish for cooking on a barbecue. Simply mix together the various ingredients that make up the marinade, place the fish in the marinade and allow it to remain in it for up to 8 hours.

Ingredients

2 to 4 Catfish Fillets
80ml Vegetable Oil
60ml Low Sodium Soy Sauce
2 Garlic Cloves Freshly Minced
2 Tablespoons Rice Wine Vinegar
2 Tablespoons Sesame Seeds
1 Tablespoon Sesame Oil
¼ Teaspoon Freshly Ground Black Pepper
¼ Teaspoon Pepper Flakes

Instructions

1. In to a resealable plastic bag place the catfish fillets.

2. In a small bowl now combine together the vegetable oil, soy sauce, garlic, rice wine

vinegar, sesame seeds, sesame oil, black pepper and pepper flakes. Then pour over the fillets in the bag and seal it. Turn the bag over several times to ensure that the catfish fillets have been well coated in the marinade before then placing the bag in the refrigerator and leaving there for 1 to 8 hours. The longer you let the fish remain in the marinade the more of its flavor will be absorbed by the fish.

3. As soon as you are ready to cook the fish then heat up the barbecue and make sure that you place the grill at a height that allows you to cook the catfish fillets on a medium to high heat.

4. Once the barbecue has heated up remove the catfish fillets from the marinade, which can now be discarded and place the fillets on the grill, which you have lightly oiled first and cook for between 12 and 13 minutes. During this time you must turn the fillets over at least once. The fish will be cooked when it easily flakes with a fork. As soon as the fish is cooked remove from heat and serve to your guests.

Recipe 15 – Barbecued Sea Bass

This is a very simple barbecue recipe for cooking sea bass. However it is best if at possible to use as fresh a fish as possible. Not only perfect for cooking at home but also at the beach.

Ingredients

500gram Fresh Sea Bass
1 Tablespoon Fresh Lemon Juice
1 Teaspoon Olive Oil
Salt & Freshly Ground Black Pepper To Taste
1 Bay Leaf

Instructions

1. In a bowl mix together the lemon juice, olive oil, salt, pepper and bay leaf. Then rub the sea bass both inside and out with this. You should be doing this whilst the barbecue is heating up.

2. As soon as the barbecue has heated up place the fish on the lightly oiled grilled about 4 to 6 inches above the heat source and cook for around 8 to 10 minutes. Halfway through

the cooking time you should turn the fish over and finish off cooking. You will know when the fish is cooked as it flakes easily with a fork.

Recipe 16 – Grilled Trout In Corn Husks

This is a recipe that will impress your guests and also is a very quick and easy way to prepare and serve trout to them.

Ingredients

4 Trout Fillets
4 Fresh Corn Husks
8 Strips Bacon
20grams Unsalted Butter
½ Teaspoon Freshly Ground Black Pepper

Kitchen Twine

Instructions

1. Check the fish over to make sure that there are no bones in the fillets. Whilst you are doing this now is the time to get the barbecue heated up.

2. Once you have checked to make sure there are no more bones in the fish you can now start making up the little corn husk packets. Place a fillet on each corn husk and then over these place two of the slices of bacon along

with 5 grams of the butter. Now close the husks up and secure them in place by wrapping some of the kitchen twine around them.

3. Once you have placed the twine around the corn husks you can place the packets on to the barbecue grill and cook for between 15 and 18 minutes or until the fish is cooked through. As soon as the fish is ready remove from heat and serve to your guests with barbecued corn on the cob and some fresh new potatoes.

Recipe 17 – Grilled Jamaican Jerk Catfish

Although relatively spicy you can add a little more of kick to yours if want by adding an additional freshly chopped jalapeno in to the seasoning mixture.

Ingredients

4 Catfish Fillets
2 Green Onions Finely Chopped
1 Jalapeno Pepper Seeded And Chopped
2 Tablespoons Brown Sugar
2 Tablespoons Worcestershire Sauce
2 Tablespoons White Wine Vinegar
1 Tablespoon Freshly Minced Ginger
1 Garlic Clove Minced
1 Teaspoon Allspice
½ Teaspoon Dried Thyme
¼ Teaspoon Salt
1/8 Teaspoon Freshly Ground Black Pepper

Instructions

1. Preheat heat the barbecue to a medium heat. Whilst the barbecue is heating up in to a bowl (large) place the onions, jalapeno pepper, brown sugar, Worcestershire sauce, white

wine vinegar, ginger, garlic, allspice, dried thyme, salt and pepper and mix thoroughly.

2. Now into the bowl add the fish and coat well before then covering the bowl and leaving the fish to marinate in the sauce for 5 to 10 minutes at room temperature.

3. After the relevant amount of time has elapsed remove the catfish fillets from the marinade and place them to one side. Don't throw away the marinade as you are going to need this.

4. Place the catfish fillets on the barbecue grill that has been lightly oiled and brush with some of the remaining marinade. Now cook for about 5 minutes before then turning the fish over. After turning the fish over you need to again brush with the marinade that is remaining and cook for a further 7 to 9 minutes. As soon as the fillets are cooked remove from the barbecue and serve with a crisp fresh green salad.

Recipe 18 – Grilled Tandoori Cod

As well as being very easy to prepare you will find that this particular recipe tastes absolutely delicious. Serve either with some freshly grilled vegetables or with some rice.

Ingredients

4 to 6 Cod Fillets Cut Into ½ Inch Chunks
240ml Plain Yogurt
60ml Olive Oil
4 Garlic Cloves Minced
2 Teaspoons Freshly Grated Ginger
2 Teaspoons Ground Cumin
2 Teaspoons Ground Coriander
1 Teaspoon Red Pepper
1 Teaspoon Turmeric
1 Teaspoon Salt

Instructions

1. In a medium size bowl combine together the yogurt, olive oil, garlic, ginger, cumin, coriander, red pepper, turmeric and salt. Once combined together well add the chunks of cod and mix again. It is important to make sure

that every piece of cod is coated well in the marinade you have just made.

2.   Now cover the bowl over and place in a refrigerator for 1 hour to let the fish absorb as much of the marinade as possible.

3.   About 15 minutes before you remove the fish from the refrigerator you should now start heating up your barbecue. Put the grill at a height of about 4 to 6 inches above the heat source so that the fish will then cook on a medium to high heat.

4.   As soon as the barbecue has heated up sufficiently you are now ready to start cooking the fish. Remove the fish from the marinade and thread on to wooden skewers that have been soaking in water for around 30 minutes and then place them on to the lightly oiled grill.

Cook for around 17 to 19 minutes turning frequently to ensure that the fish doesn't get burnt. When the flesh of the code turns opaque you can now remove from the heat and serve.

Recipe 19 – Grilled Mustard & Miso Sea Bass

This particular recipe requires you to use white miso paste that is much sweeter and milder than the dark versions. When you allow the sea bass to marinade in the miso, rice wine and mustard sauce it help to make the fish much tenderer and taste more delicious.

Ingredients

4 Sea Bass Fillets each weighing About 140 to 170grams
6 Green Onions Trimmed
80ml White Miso Paste
3 Tablespoons Rice Vinegar
2 Tablespoons Japanese Rice Wine (Mirin)
2 Tablespoons Toasted Sesame Seeds
3 Teaspoons Sugar
2 Teaspoons Water
1 Garlic Clove Minced
1 Teaspoon Dijon Mustard
1 Teaspoon Soy Sauce
Olive Oil
Salt
Freshly Ground Black Pepper

Instructions

1. Whilst the barbecue is heating up in to a bowl mix together the water and mustard until they are mixed thoroughly.

2. Now into a small saucepan place the miso, vinegar, mirin, soy sauce, garlic, sugar and mustard mixture and place pan on to a medium heat. Whisk the mixture whilst heating until it turns smooth, this should take between 3 to 5 minutes to happen. Once the mixture has turned smooth remove from heat and brush the sauce over the fish and also brush the green onions with some olive oil. Sprinkle the fish and onions with salt and pepper to taste.

3. Now place the fish on to the barbecue grill which has been lightly oiled and cook on either side for 4 to 5 minutes or the flesh inside turns opaque in color.

4. Next you need to cook the fish for a further 2 minutes on either side and whilst this is happening you should place the green onions on the grill to cook as well.

You are now ready to remove the fish and onions from the barbecue to serve to your guests. Place each fish on a clean plate with the onions and a small amount of the miso sauce you have left over and sprinkle over some of the toasted sesame seeds.

Recipe 20 – Sea Bass Kebabs

If you want to prepare sea bass quickly and easily this is the perfect barbecue recipe to use. They are suitable for any kind of barbecue party you are going to be having.

Ingredients

680grams Sea Bass Cut Into ½ Inch Chunks
60ml Fresh Lemon Juice
60ml Olive Oil
2 Garlic Cloves Minced
1 Teaspoon Dried Oregano
¼ Teaspoon Salt
¼ Teaspoon Freshly Ground Black Pepper

Instructions

1. In a large bowl mix together the lemon juice, olive oil, garlic, oregano, salt and pepper. Once thoroughly combined together add in the chunks of sea bass and then cover the bowl and place in the refrigerator to marinate for 1 to 2 hours.

2. About 15 minutes before you remove the sea bass from the refrigerator you should start

warming up the barbecue. You will need to cook the kebabs on a very high heat. If you are going to be using wooden skewers then make sure that these have been soaking in water for no less than an hour, as this will then prevent them from burning when placed on the barbecue.

3. As you remove each piece of fish from the marinade thread them on to the skewers and place to one side ready for cooking. Don't discard any leftover marinade, as you will be using this later on when cooking the fish.

4. As soon as the barbecue is hot enough you can place the kebabs on the grill. Make sure that you have lightly oiled the grill first to prevent the fish kebabs from sticking to it and cook them for between 5 and 7 minutes. As well as turning the kebabs over frequently to prevent them from burning also baste them with any marinade that is left over. As soon as the kebabs are ready serve.

Recipe 21 – Grilled Thai Red Snapper Packets

This recipe allows you to cook red snapper on your barbecue without leaving any mess to clear up afterwards.

Ingredients

4 Red Snapper Fillets (140 to 170grams)
1 Carrot Julienne
1 Green Onion Minced

32grams Fresh Cilantro
3 Tablespoons Fresh Lime Juice
2 Garlic Cloves Minced
1 Tablespoon Fish Sauce
1 Tablespoon Olive Oil
1 Teaspoon Freshly Minced Ginger
Aluminum Foil

Instructions

1. Start the barbecue is up so it is ready for placing the packets containing the red snapper on to cook.

2. Whilst the barbecue is heating up in a small bowl mix together the fish sauce, olive oil, ginger, lime juice, sugar and garlic.

3. On to four separate pieces of aluminum foil you place one of the four red snapper fillets (skin side down) and pour over some of the mixture you have just made. Then sprinkle over the top of this some of the carrots, cilantro and green onion. Then bring up the sides of the aluminum to seal the fish inside. But don't secure the packets too tightly as you need to allow some of the steam produced as the fish cooks to escape.

4. As soon as the barbecue has heated up place the Thai red snapper packets on the grill and cook for between 8 and 10 minutes. Once this time has elapsed remove from the barbecue and then cut open the packets with a pair of scissors and serve without removing them from the aluminum foil on a clean plate.

Recipe 22 – Moroccan Grilled Fish Kebabs

This is very simple dish to prepare but provides the fish you use with lots of flavor.

Ingredients

680grams White Fish Fillets Cut Into Chunks
32grams Red Onion Chopped
80ml Olive Oil
2 Tablespoons Fresh Cilantro Finely Chopped
3 Tablespoons Fresh Lemon Juice
½ Teaspoon Paprika
½ Teaspoon Salt
¼ Teaspoon Freshly Ground Black Pepper
¼ Teaspoon Chilli Powder
2 Garlic Cloves Minced

Wooden Skewers which have been soaked in water for at least 30 minutes.

Instructions

1. Cut the fillets of fish into chunks measuring an inch each and place them in a resealable plastic bag.

2. Now in to a bowl place the onion, olive oil, cilantro, lemon juice, paprika, salt, pepper, chilli powder and minced garlic and stir well to ensure that the ingredients are mixed thoroughly together. Now pour this mixture into the same bag as the fish. Then close the bag and turn it over or shake until all pieces of fish have been coated in the marinade you have just made. Once you have done this place the sealed bag in to a refrigerator and leave there for between 2 and 4 hours.

3. When it comes to cooking the fish remove from the bag discarding any marinade that remains and thread each chunk of fish on to the skewers you have been soaking in water. Once you have thread each skewer with fish you should now lightly oil the grill on your preheated barbecue and place the skewers on to it.

You should be cooking the fish kebabs on a medium to high heat for between 8 and 10 minutes making sure that you turn them over occasionally to prevent them from burning. As soon as they have cooked you should remove them from the barbecue and serve to your guests immediately.

Recipe 23 – Grilled Fish Cakes

It is possible to cook fish cakes on a grill but you do need to be careful when doing so.

Ingredients

450grams White Fish Fillets
1 Onion Chopped
6 Cashew Nuts
1 Teaspoon Chilli Powder
½ Teaspoon Tumeric
1 Tablespoon Freshly Chopped Lemon Grass
1 Teaspoon Freshly Chopped Mint
½ Teaspoon Freshly Grated Black Pepper
1 Tablespoon Sugar
120ml Coconut Milk
1 Tablespoon Coriander
Salt To Taste
Banana Leafs For Cooking The Fish Cakes In

Instructions

1. The first thing you should do before you cut the fish fillets into small pieces is to make sure that there no bones inside them.

2.   After cutting the fish fillets into small pieces mix them together with the onion, nuts, chilli powder, turmeric, lemon grass, mint, black pepper, sugar, coconut milk, coriander and salt in a food processor until they form a smooth mixture.

3.   Before you can place any of the fish cake mixture on to a piece of banana leaf measuring 6 inches square they leaves need to be boiled in water for about a minute as this will help to soften them up and make them more pliable to use. As soon as the banana leaves are ready place 2 tablespoons of the fish cake mixture on to each one and then fold the leaves over. To keep the leaves securely in place pierce through the areas where they come together with a toothpick. You should be doing this whilst the barbecue is heating up.

4.   As soon as the barbecue has heated place the banana leaves with the fish cake mixture inside on to the barbecue and cook on a high heat for 5 minutes. It is important that halfway through this time you turn the fish cakes over to ensure that they are cooked evenly. Once the fish cakes are ready serve to your guests still encased in the banana leaves.

Recipe 24 – Tarragon Fish With Vegetables

Wrapping up the fish with the vegetables and tarragon help to add more flavor to this dish. Plus you won't make as much mess when cooking them because the fish and other ingredients are wrapped up.

Ingredients

2 x 170grams Fish Fillets (You May Want To Give Orange Roughy A Try)
½ Zucchini Cut Into Julienne Strips
½ Small Red Bell Pepper Cut Into Thin Strips
32grams Sliced Red Onion
1 Carrot Cut Into Julienne Strips
1 Tablespoon Canola Oil
2 Tablespoons Freshly Chopped Tarragon (If you cannot get hold of fresh tarragon use ¾ Teaspoon of Dried Tarragon Instead)
1 Tablespoon Butter

Instructions

1. Whilst the barbecue is heating up in a frying pan place the oil and cook the vegetables for about 2 to 3 minutes on a

medium to high heat. Then place to one side, as you will need them in a minute.

2. Next take too large pieces of aluminum foil and on to these place the fish fillets then on top of these place ½ tablespoon of the butter, half the vegetables and half of the tarragon. Then tightly wrap the foil around each piece and place on the grill of the barbecue.

3. Grill each piece of fish on a medium heat for between 12 and 18 minutes. How long you cook them for will depend on how thick each fish fillet is. The thicker the fillet then the longer they will need to remain on the barbecue.

It is important that after removing the packets from the barbecue that you open them carefully as the steam released can be extremely hot and can cause burns.

Recipe 25 – Italian Style Trout

The stuffing of the trout with the olives and shallots adds even more flavor to what is a very tasty fish. Make sure that you cook these on a very high heat and don't allow them to remain on the barbecue for too long.

Ingredients

4 Trout (Heads Removed, Boned And Butterflied)
4 Tablespoons Butter
32grams Black Olives Which Have Been Coarsely Chopped
2 Tablespoons Pernod (Or Other Liquorice Flavored Liqueur)
2 Tablespoons Olive Oil
1 Tablespoon Freshly Chopped Parsley
1 Small Chopped Shallot
1 Teaspoon Salt
1 Teaspoon Freshly Chopped Chives
½ Teaspoon Freshly Ground Black Pepper
1/8 Teaspoon Freshly Ground Black Pepper

Instructions

1. Sprinkle both sides of the fish with the salt, ½ teaspoon black pepper and Pernod. Now cover and leave the fish to stand for around 30 minutes at room temperature. Whilst this is happening now would be a good time to get the barbecue started.

2. Whilst the fish is left to one side you now need to make up the mixture, which you will then stuff the fish fillets with. In a food processor place the shallots and olives and process them until they are finely chopped. Now to this mixture add the butter, chives, parsley and the 1/8 teaspoon freshly ground black pepper and again turn the food processor on to blend all these ingredients together well. Once the mixture is ready stuff it inside the fillets of trout and fold the opening closed. If you want you can prevent the fillet from opening again by securing it with a toothpick.

3. As soon as the barbecue has heated up place the trout fillets on to the grill and cook on a medium to high heat for 8 minutes on each side. As soon as the cooking time has been completed remove from heat and serve to your guests on clean plates with a crisp fresh green salad.

Recipe 26 – Perch With Sage

This is a really wonderful little recipe to try if you want to grill several perch at once.

Ingredients

2 x 340grams Perch (Scaled)
2 Slices of Zucchini
3 Roma Tomatoes
1 Tablespoon Olive Oil
10 Sprigs of Fresh Sage

Instructions

1.   Whilst the barbecue is heating up make around 4 slits into the flesh of the perch on each side. Now coat them with oil and insert sprigs of sage into them.

2.   Once the barbecue has heated up place the perch on to the oiled grill and cook for around 4 minutes on each side. As you are about to turn the fish over you should now add the zucchini and tomatoes on to the grill and cook these.

3. As soon as everything has cooked remove everything from the barbecue. To serve the fish remove the sprigs of sage and then stuff them with the tomatoes and zucchini.

Recipe 27 – Sweet & Sour Halibut

The rich thick sauce that you will eventually pour over the halibut steaks is the same one that you marinated the fish in originally. However it is best to reserve some of the marinate to make the sauce as you don't want it to become contaminated by the fish. This sauce provides the halibut steaks with a great deal of flavor without being too much hassle to create.

Ingredients

4 x Halibut Steaks (Weighing About 340grams Each)

1 Red and Green Bell Pepper
2 Green Onions Cut Into 2 Inch Strips
60ml Water
55grams Brown Sugar
3 Tablespoons Cider Vinegar
3 Tablespoons Tomato Ketchup
1 Tablespoon Soy Sauce
2 Garlic Cloves Minced
¾ Teaspoon Freshly Grated Ginger

Instructions

1. Coat the grill on your barbecue with oil and then turn it on so it can start heating up.

2. Take the bell peppers and cut them in half and remove the seeds then set to one side for use later on.

3. In a bowl place the brown sugar, water, cider vinegar, tomato ketchup, soy sauce, garlic and ginger and mix well together. Remove around 60ml of the sauce you have just made and set aside for later.

4. With the rest of the sauce you have just made dip each of the halibut steaks into it making sure that both sides of the fish have

been evenly coated in it and again set to one side.

5. By now the grill should have heated up and you should place the bell peppers on them to cook. Place the peppers on the grill with the skin side down and cook until the skin begins to blacken. Remove once the skin starts to blacken and peel it away from the rest of the pepper. Once the skin has been removed cut them peppers into thin strips.

6. Now place the halibut steaks on the grill and cook until they are done the flesh should start to turn opaque in color. Once the steaks are cooked place each one on a clean plate then top with some of the slices of the bell peppers and the green onions before then pouring over equal amounts of the sauce that you put aside earlier.

Recipe 28 – Halibut & Red Pepper Kebabs

Halibut is one of the least expensive fishes you can buy today. However by putting the fish onto skewers with peppers and onions you can ensure that you are able to feed more people with only a small amount of the fish.

Ingredients

680grams Halibut Steaks Cut Into 1 Inch Chunks
1 Large Bell Pepper Cut Into 1 Inch Squares
1 Large Red Onion Cut Into 1 Inch Squares
120ml Fresh Lime Juice
4 Tablespoons Olive Oil
3 Tablespoons Fresh Finely Chopped Cilantro
2 Tablespoons Sugar
1 ½ Teaspoons Serrano Pepper Minced (It is important that you wear gloves when dealing with this type of pepper)

Instructions

1. In a small bowl place the lime juice, 2 tablespoons of olive oil, sugar, Serrano pepper and the sugar and combine well together until all the sugar has dissolved. Now leave this to

one side for around an hour so that all the flavors blend together.

2. Whilst the sauce is blending you should now be turning the barbecue on so that it can heat up ready to start cooking the halibut, pepper and onion kebabs.

3. To make the kebabs you should thread on to each one alternate pieces of the halibut, pepper and onion until they are all used up. Metal skewers can be used however if you intend to use wooden ones make sure that they have been soaking in some water for at least an hour to ensure that they don't burn when placed on the barbecue.

4. Before you place the kebabs on the grill brush them all over with the remaining olive oil and cook on a high heat for about 1 ½ minutes on all sides so you should be cooking them for a total of around 6 minutes. You will know that the halibut is cooked as it will have turned opaque and will be flaky through the middle.

5. After removing the kebabs from the grill onto a clean plate now serve them with the sauce you made earlier alongside.

Recipe 29 – Fish Roll Ups

A very traditional Australian recipe you may want to try out this summer.

Ingredients

100grams Smoked Fish
240ml Milk
6 Slices of Buttered Bread
22grams Grated Cheese
3 Tablespoons Butter
3 Tablespoons Flour
1 Teaspoon Lemon Juice (Fresh Is Best)
1 Teaspoon Freshly Chopped Parsley
½ Teaspoon Worcestershire Sauce
¼ Teaspoon Salt
¼ Teaspoon Freshly Ground Black Pepper

Instructions

1. Whilst the barbecue is heating up flake the smoked fish and melt the butter in a saucepan to which you then add the flour, pepper, salt and parsley. Cook this mixture until it begins to boil then very slowly add the milk and then continue cook for a further two minutes. Now add the Worcestershire sauce, cheese, lemon

juice and the flaked smoked fish. Mix all the ingredients together well.

2. Now take this mixture and spread it over the unbuttered side of the bread and roll each one up and secure them using a toothpick.

3. Once you have made up each fish roll place them on the barbecue grill, which you can lightly oil, and cook for around 2 to 3 minutes. During this time make sure that you turn them over once and then serve immediately to your waiting guests

Recipe 30 – Grilled Snapper In A Banana Leaf

This particular method of cooking not only helps to keep the fish together but also helps to steam it to perfection, but still allows some of the smoky flavor to permeate through to the fish also. Plus this method also allows you to add anything you want to the packet to bring out the flavor of the fish even more.

Ingredients

900grams Snapper
2 Tablespoons Freshly Chopped Coriander Root
1 ½ Tablespoons Soy Sauce
1 Tablespoon Freshly Crushed Ginger
2 Garlic Cloves Minced
1 Teaspoon Freshly Ground Black Pepper
Vegetable Oil
Banana Leaf
String

Instructions

1. Into a food processor place the garlic, ginger, black pepper and coriander root and

blend together so that it forms a paste. Then add the soy sauce and continue to blend until all the ingredients become well combined. Now set this mixture to one side.

2. Next you should rinse the snapper and then pat it dry with some paper towels. Once you have done this take the sauce you made earlier and rub it all over the surface of the fish and place the fish to one side for 30 minutes. It is now that you should be starting your barbecue up so that it has reached the required temperature for cooking the fish on.

3. Once the 30 minutes have elapsed take the snapper and place it on to the banana leaf. It is important that the leaves you use are large enough to completely cover the fish. However if you cannot get large ones then it is perfectly to cut the fish into pieces that will fit easily inside the leaves you do have.

But before you do wrap the fish in the leaves make sure that you have washed them thoroughly. Also they need to be blanched in hot water for a number of seconds as this will help to make the soft and so much easier to wrap around the fish.

After the banana leaves have been blanched you should remove the thick spine from them with a pair of kitchen scissors. Then place them on a work surface shiny side facing downwards.

Then you must brush vegetable oil all over the leaf facing towards you, which will then come into contact with the fish. Once you have done this you can place the fish on to and then wrap the leaf around it. To help keep the leaf around the fish when cooking secure it in place either with a skewer or toothpicks.

4.   After wrapping the snapper in the banana leaf you can now place it on the barbecue to cook. Cook it on a medium heat so place the grill around 4 to 6 inches above the heat source and cook on each side for between 8 and 10 minutes. You need to keep an eye on the fish as it is cooking to ensure that the banana leaf doesn't become burnt. Although it may start to blacken in areas you don't want the heat to burn right through the leaf.

5. After 16 minutes remove the packages from the barbecue and very gently open them to see whether the fish is cooked or not. You will know when the fish is cooked because it is

opaque in appearance and flakes easily with a fork. If you notice that the fish isn't cooked then securely wrap back in the banana leaf and place on the barbecue again for another couple of minutes.

When it comes to serving this dish it is best to allow the fish to remain enclosed in the banana leaf and open it when you reach the table.

Recipe 31 – South Western Mahi Mahi

This is the perfect recipe to use if you want to serve Mexican style food for your guests at your next barbecue. You can use this particular recipe to make some amazing fish tacos.

Ingredients

6 x 170grams Mahi Mahi Fish Fillets (If you cannot get hold of this fish then use Halibut fillets instead)
40grams Freshly Chopped Cilantro
60ml Fresh Lemon Juice
2 Tablespoons Olive Oil
1 Tablespoon Honey
3 Garlic Cloves Minced
1 Teaspoon Hot Chilli Powder (Optional)
Salt and Freshly Ground Black Pepper To Taste

Instructions

1. In a bowl combine well together the cilantro, lemon juice, olive oil, honey, garlic, salt and pepper. Plus the hot chilli powder if you want to add a little kick to this dish. Then set to one side.

Samantha Michaels

2. Now into a resealable bag or on a shallow baking dish place the fish fillets and pour over the sauce you made earlier.

Remember to turn the fish over so that all sides are coated in the marinade and leave if the refrigerator to marinate for 30 minutes. Whilst the fish is marinating in the refrigerator you should be lighting your barbecue so that it is ready then for cooking the fish once you take it out of the refrigerator.

3. To cook the fish remove from the marinade and place on the barbecue directly over the heat sauce and then cook on each side for 3 to 4 minutes or until the fish is cooked through. To check to see if it is done see if the fish flakes easily with a fork and has turned opaque through out.

Recipe 32 – Grilled Shark

Shark actually has a great flavor and the sauce in which you marinate the fish helps to enhance rather than overpower its flavor.

Ingredients

6 Shark Steaks
120ml Soy Sauce
60ml Tomato Ketchup
120ml Fresh Orange Juice
40grams Freshly Chopped Parsley
2 Tablespoons Fresh Lemon Juice
2 Garlic Cloves Minced
1/3 Tablespoon Freshly Ground Pepper

Instructions

1.   In a bowl combine together the garlic, pepper, soy sauce, orange juice, tomato ketchup, chopped parsley and lemon juice.

2.   Take the shark steaks and place them in a shallow baking dish and pour the sauce you have just made over them. It is important that you turn the steaks over to ensure that all sides of them are coated in the sauce, which you are

going to be marinating them in. Now cover the dish and place in the refrigerator for 2 hours.

3. When it comes time to cook the shark steaks make sure that the grill on the barbecue has been lightly oiled first to prevent them from sticking to the surface. As soon as the barbecue has heated up remove the steaks from the marinate and place them on the grill keeping any leftover marinate in the dish for use later.

4. Grill the shark steaks over a high heat for 6 minutes on each side or until when tested with a fork the fish flakes easily. Throughout the time the shark steaks are cooking make sure that you baste them regularly with the remainder of the sauce you marinated them in earlier.

Recipe 33 – Grilled Catfish

Not only is this a quick and easy way to cook catfish. But adding the sauce whilst cooking adds even more flavor to it.

Ingredients

450grams Catfish Fillet
3 Garlic Cloves Crushed
2 Tablespoons Lemon Juice (Fresh If Possible)
1 Tablespoon Balsamic Vinegar
1 Teaspoon Soy Sauce
2 Sprigs Fresh Rosemary
1 Teaspoon Cayenne Pepper

Instructions

1. Whilst the barbecue is heating up place the catfish fillet on to a piece of aluminum foil that is large enough that when you fold the edges up it turns into a makeshift pan.

2. Now place the fish in the aluminum foil on to the barbecue and them pour over the other ingredients and let the catfish fillet cook them until it is done. On average the fish should be cooked in about 4 to 9 minutes depending on

how hot the barbecue is and what the weather is like. It is important that you watch the fish carefully whilst it is cooking otherwise it could become over cooked very easily.

You will know when the fish is cooked because the edges of it start to turn up and become crispy. But don't rely on this solely for telling you that the fish is cooked you should check to see if the middle of the catfish fillet has turned opaque.

Recipe 34 – Spicy Tuna Steaks

When it comes to cooking tuna steaks on a barbecue make sure that you do so on a very high heat. Also use the best quality steaks you can, as these will only require warming through to the middle.

Ingredients

6 Small Tuna Steaks (Weighing Around 170grams Each)
80ml Olive Oil
80ml Lemon Juice (Fresh Would Be Best)
4 Tablespoons Chopped Cilantro Leaves
3 Garlic Cloves Minced
3 Shallots Minced
2 Teaspoons Cayenne Pepper
2 Teaspoons Ground Cumin
1 Teaspoon Salt

Instructions

1. In a bowl combine together well the lemon juice, olive oil, and 3 tablespoons of the cilantro leaves, garlic, shallots, cumin, cayenne pepper and salt.

2. Now into a large resealable bag you place the tuna steaks and then pour the sauce you have just made over them. Make sure that you turn the bag over several times to ensure the sauce coats the steaks evenly then place in the refrigerator for 1 hour to allow them to marinate in the sauce.

3. About 15 minutes before you remove the tuna steaks from the refrigerator you should start up your barbecue so it is heated up correctly for cooking the steaks on it.

4. Just before you take the steaks out of the marinade after removing from the refrigerator lightly oil the grill on your barbecue and then place the tuna steaks on them. Make sure the grill is placed as close to the heat source as possible as you need to cook the steaks on a high heat.

5. You should cook each side of the tuna steaks for around 4 to 5 minutes or until you feel they are cooked to the way people enjoy eating this type of fish. Once they are cooked remove from the barbecue place on clean plates and sprinkle with the remaining cilantro and then serve.

Recipe 35 – Asian Jerk Red Snapper

As well as using jerk seasoning this particular recipe also uses an Asian style baste to help bring out even more of the wonderful flavor of this particular fish.

Ingredients

2 Whole Red Snapper (Weighing About 900grams Each)
4 Green Onions Diced
4 Garlic Cloves Minced
60ml Lemon Juice
Zest Of Two Lemons
2 Tablespoons Jerk Rub
2 Tablespoons Olive Oil
2 Tablespoons Soy Sauce

Instructions

1. In a small bowl combine together 2 minced garlic cloves, scallions, lemon zest and 1 tablespoon Jerk rub. Then rub it all over the insides of the cleaned out red snapper.

2. Now into another bowl you should combine together the other 1 tablespoon jerk rub along

with the rest of the garlic, the lemon juice, the soy sauce and olive oil and place to one side. It is important that before you start making up the above you actually turn the barbecue on so it will then be ready for cooking the fish on.

3. As soon as the barbecue has heated up place the red snapper on to the grill about 4 to 6 inches above the heat source so it cooks on a medium to high heat. Let the fish cook on each side for 8 to 10 minutes and whilst this is happening baste frequently with the lemon, soy sauce and jerk rub sauce.

Recipe 36 – Grilled Fresh Sardines

This recipe helps to turn what is quite a humble fish into something a little special. Plus it is also good for your health as it helps to reduce "bad cholesterol" levels.

Ingredients

8 Medium Sized Whole Fresh Sardines
(These should be gutted, and then rinsed inside and out before then being patted dry with a paper towel).
1 ½ Tablespoons Extra Virgin Olive Oil
¾ Teaspoon Coarse Salt
¼ Teaspoon Freshly Ground Black Pepper
1 Garlic Clove Peeled
6 Inch Baguette Cut Into 16 Thin Slices Diagonally

Instructions

1. Brush both sides of the sardines with 1 tablespoon of the extra virgin olive oil and thin sprinkle over them 1/2 teaspoon of salt and 1/8 teaspoon of the freshly ground black pepper. Whilst you are doing this heat up the barbecue.

2. Once the barbecue is hot enough lightly oil the surface of the grill and them place the sardines on to it and cook them on a medium to high heat. Cook each sardine for 2 minutes on each side.

3. Halfway through cooking the sardines you should also be cooking the slices of baguette that you will be serving with the fish.

But before placing the baguette slices on the barbecue first rub each side of them with the garlic and brush them with the rest of the olive oil. Then sprinkle with the salt and pepper that is left over. Cook each side of the bread for 1 minute or until they turn crisp.

4. As soon as everything is cooked place the sardines and bread on to a clean plate and serve with some lemon wedges to your guests.

Recipe 37 – Grilled Squid With Ginger, Celery & Apple Salad

This really does give a kick to this particular recipe and also helps to counteract some of the heat generated by the ginger.

Ingredients

8 Squid Bodies (Rinsed and Dried)
1 Garlic Clove Minced
3 Tablespoons White Or Light Miso Paste
3 Tablespoons Sake
2 Teaspoons Mirin
1 Tablespoon Soy Sauce
1 Tablespoon Oyster Sauce

For The Salad

2 Teaspoons Freshly Grated Ginger
1 ½ Teaspoons Cider Vinegar
Juice of 1 Lime
½ Teaspoon Sugar
3 Tablespoons Vegetable or Canola Oil
5 Stalks of Celery Halved Lengthways then Sliced Diagonally into 2 ½ inch pieces
1 Tart Apple (Granny Smith is Ideal) Peeled then Cut Into Matchstick Size Pieces

2 Green Onions Halved Lengthways Then Slice Into 2 ½ inch Matchsticks (Use the white and pale green parts only)
110grams Sunflower Sprouts
1 Serrano Chilli Halved Lengthways, Seeds Removed And Thinly Sliced Crosswise
1 Teaspoon Black Sesame Seeds
Coarse Salt to Taste

Instructions

1. In a saucepan mix together the garlic, white or light miso paste, sake, mirin, soy sauce and oyster sauce to make a marinade. You need to cook this sauce over a medium to high heat for around 3 minutes, making sure that you stir it continuously. After the 3 minutes have elapsed remove from heat and place in a bowl to cool slightly.

2. You now need to tenderize the squid to do this you need to pound both sides of it with a kitchen mallet a few times. Then cut along the seam of the squid with a sharp knife so you can open it up and lightly score the inside at ¼ inch intervals. After doing this add the squid to the marinade and leave it to stand for 20 minutes.

3. Whilst the squid is marinating in the sauce you can now make the dressing to go with the salad that you will serve with the grilled squid. First of all you need to whisk together the ginger, lime juice, vinegar, sugar and salt and add the oil to it very slowly until the liquid becomes emulsified.

4. To cook the squid on the barbecue you need to make sure that it is preheated to a medium to high heat. When the barbecue is heated up you can now cook the squid. You will need to use something to put on top of the squid as it is cooking lining a skillet with aluminum foil and put something like bricks in it should help.

5. Before you place the squid on the grill sprinkle the scored sides of the squid with salt and then place them facing down on to the grill. It is a good idea to lightly oil the grill first before placing the squid on it to prevent them from sticking.

Once you have placed the squid on the grill place the weighted skillet on top and let them cook for about 1 ½ minutes. Once the squid is cooked remove and cut into ¾ inch pieces.

6. To finish off take the apple, celery, green onions, sprouts and chilli into a bowl and pour over 3 tablespoons of the dressing made earlier. Toss the ingredients so that they are all coated in the dressing then place some on to a clean plate with some of the squid on top before then sprinkling over this some sesame seeds.

Recipe 38 – Monkfish & Prawn Kebabs With Tomato Salsa

These kebabs taste really wonderful when served with a Mexican style tomato sauce.

Ingredients

700grams Monkfish Tail
100grams about 4 Large Raw Tiger Prawns or 8 to 12 Smaller Ones
1 Garlic Clove Crushed
1 Teaspoon Ginger Puree or Freshly Grated Ginger
1 Green Chilli (Deseeded and Finely Chopped)
1 Tablespoon Sunflower or Ground Nut Oil
Salt and Freshly Ground Black Pepper To Taste

Salsa

500grams Plum Tomatoes
2 Teaspoons Coriander Seeds
1 Green Chilli (Deseeded and Finely Chopped)
1 Garlic Clove Crushed
1 Stalk Lemongrass (Outer Leaves Removed Then Finely Sliced)
Juice of 1 Lime

Wedges of Lime To Serve With Dish
Instructions

1. Rinse the monkfish in cold water and then pat dry with paper towels. Remove any grey membrane and then cut the flesh away from the backbone cartilage so you have two long pieces. Then cut each piece into equal size chunks. You should aim to get between 8 and 12 chunks from each piece.

2. Next you need to peel the prawns if you can leave the tails on and just remove the legs and heads. Now run a sharp knife along the back of each prawn and pull out the dark thread running through him or her. Then rinse them in cold water then pat dry and put to one side for use later as with the monkfish.

NB: It would be a good idea to put the monkfish and prawns in the refrigerator until needed.

3. Now you are ready to start making the marinade for the kebabs. To do this mix the garlic, chilli, ginger and oil in a bowl and then to this add the monkfish and prawns and mix all ingredients together well. Now cover the

top of the bowl with cling film and place in the refrigerator for 1 hour. Whilst the fish and prawns are marinating take your wooden skewers and place them in some water to soak.

4. Whilst the monkfish and prawns are marinating you can begin making the salsa. First off you need to cover the tomatoes with boiling water and then leave them like this for one minute. After a minute has passed remove the tomatoes from the water and peel away the skin and cut in half so that you can remove the seeds. Now cut each half of the tomato into chunky puree. Unfortunately you will have to do this by hand rather than using a food processor.

5. Now place the chunks of tomato into a bowl and into this mix the chilli, garlic, lime juice and lemongrass. Then add a little salt and pepper to taste. Cover the bowl over and place in the refrigerator ready for when you want to serve the kebabs.

6. To cook the kebabs you need to place them on the barbecue grill on a medium to high heat and cook each one for between 3 to 4 minutes on both sides. You can tell when the kebabs are ready, as the prawns will have turned a

pink color and feel much firmer. You should have threaded onto each skewer chunks of monkfish and 1, 2 or 3 prawns (dependent on their   size).

Recipe 39 – Skewered Swordfish With Charred Courgettes

Swordfish is ideally suited to being cooked on skewers because the flesh is so firm. Serve this particular dish with some warm focaccia bread.

Ingredients

500grams Swordfish Steaks Cut Into 2cm Chunks
3 Lemons
3 Tablespoon Olive Oil
1 Garlic Clove Crushed
15grams Fresh Basil Chopped
500grams Small Courgettes Trimmed

Instructions

1.   Whilst four long wooden skewers are soaking in water you need to cut the swordfish up into 2cm chunks. To do this you first need to cut away the skin. As the skin is quite thick you need to use a very sharp knife.

2.   In a bowl grate the zest from one of the lemons and add to this the juice of it along

with the olive oil and garlic and then add to it the finely chopped up basil leaves then mix well together. As for the other two lemons you now need to cut these into 8 wedges.

3. Next cut the courgettes in half lengthways and then score the white flesh with the tip of a sharp knife so a criss-cross pattern is formed on them. Then lightly brush with some of the marinade you have just made and set to one side for cooking on the barbecue later.

4. Now into the marinade you need to put the chunks of swordfish and mix well together before then placing to one side for them to marinate in the sauce for between 5 and 10 minutes. Whilst the swordfish is marinating in the sauce now is the time to turn on or light your barbecue.

5. As soon as the marinating time has elapsed you are now ready to make up the kebabs on to each skewer thread chunks of swordfish along with the lemon wedges in an alternate pattern. Then sprinkle both the kebabs and courgettes with some coarsely ground black pepper and place all items on to the barbecue grill, which has been lightly oiled.

6. Cook both the kebabs and courgettes for between 10 and 15 minutes, making sure that you turn the kebabs over occasionally to ensure that the fish is cooked right through. The same also goes for the courgettes. It is important that whilst the kebabs are cooking that you also baste them regularly with any marinade you have left over. Once the kebabs and courgettes are cooked serve to guests on clean plates along with the warm focaccia bread.

Recipe 40 – Rosemary Salmon Burgers

You may find it hard to believe but this burgers hold up extremely well when cooked on a barbecue. If you can use a good fillet of wild salmon to make the burgers from. Once cooked serve the burgers in a roll with some lettuce and tomato and a mustard and horseradish sauce.

Ingredients

1Kg King Salmon Fillet (Skinned and Bones Removed)
100grams Dried Breadcrumbs
80grams Minced Red Onion
1 Tablespoon Dijon Mustard
2 Teaspoons Horseradish (Freshly Grated If Possible)
2 Eggs (That Have Been Lightly Beaten)
1 Tablespoon Fresh Rosemary Minced
½ Teaspoon Salt
½ Teaspoon Freshly Ground Black Pepper
2 Tablespoons Olive Oil

Instructions

1. You need to cut the salmon into strips crossways and then chopping these up until the fish has become well minced. As you do chop the fish up look out for any bones and remove these.

2. Now into a large bowl place the minced salmon, breadcrumbs, red onion, mustard, horseradish and eggs. Then season this mixture with the salt and pepper and rosemary and combine them all together. Now place the mixture in the refrigerator to chill for at least 30 minutes. Whilst the salmon mixture is chilling you should now get your barbecue going and place the grill which you will have oiled just before you start cooking around 4 to 6 inches above the heat source. This is because you will be cooking the burgers on a medium to high heat.

3. After removing the salmon mixture from the refrigerator form it into 8 burger patter and then lightly coat each one with some olive oil. Then place each patty on the barbecue and cook for between 4 and 5 minutes on each side. As soon as the burgers are cooked serve on a bun with lettuce and tomato and pot of mustard and horseradish beside them.

Recipe 41 – Fast Fish Kebabs

Even though this recipe allows you to cook the fish quickly you will need to allow plenty of time for the fish to marinate. At least 2 hours should be sufficient time. If you can use any fish with firm flesh to make your kebabs from. Swordfish is ideal.

Ingredients

750grams Firm Fish Fillets
2 Tablespoons Olive Oil
1 Garlic Clove Finely Chopped
1 Tablespoon Fresh Coriander Chopped
1 Teaspoon Ground Cumin
1 Teaspoon Lemon Juice (Fresh If Possible)
Salt and Freshly Ground Black Pepper To Taste

Instructions

1. In a bowl combine together the olive oil, garlic, coriander, cumin, lemon juice, salt and pepper, then place to one side, as this is the marinade for the fish.

2. Now take the fish fillets and cut these in to 3cm size cubes and combine with the sauce you made earlier. Now place the covered bowl into a refrigerator for several hours. Whilst the fish is marinating make sure that you stir it occasionally.

3. Just before you are about to start threading the fish cubes on to wooden skewers that have been soaking in water for at least 30 minutes you should get the barbecue going.

4. It is important that before you thread the cubes of fish on to the skewers you drain them well first and also make sure that the grill on the barbecue has been oiled. Now place the skewers on the barbecue and cook each kebab for between 6 and 8 minutes turning them occasionally and also basting them with any leftover marinade. The fish is cooked through when the flesh has turned opaque and the exterior is a light brown color.

Once the kebabs are cooked serve them with a crisp green salad and some lemon wedges.

Recipe 42 – Barbecued Halibut Steaks

Although this is a very simple fish dish for cooking on the barbecue it tastes extremely delicious.

Ingredients

450grams Halibut Steak
30grams Butter
2 Tablespoons Dark Brown Soft Sugar
1 Tablespoon Lemon Juice
2 Teaspoons Soy Sauce
½ Teaspoon Freshly Ground Black Pepper

Instructions

1. Place in a small saucepan over a medium heat the butter, sugar, garlic, lemon juice, soy sauce and pepper. Stir this mixture occasionally and remove from heat as soon as all the sugar has dissolved.

2. Lightly oil your preheated barbecue with some oil and just before you place the halibut steaks on to it lightly brush each side with the sauce you made earlier. Cook each side of the fish for about 5 minutes or until the flesh of

the fish can be flaked easily with a fork. Whilst the fish is cooking make sure that you keep basting with the sauce.

3. Once the fish is cooked serve to your guests on a plate with some warm new potatoes and a crisp green salad. Otherwise you may want to consider serving the fish with some rice.

Chapter 2 – Barbecue Shellfish Recipes

Recipe 1 – Grilled King Crab Legs

Of all the recipes we provide in this book this really is the simplest among them.

Ingredients
450grams King Crab Legs Per Person
2 Tablespoons Olive Oil
2 Tablespoons Melted Butter

Instructions

1. Preheat the barbecue and place the grill around 6 inches above the heat source as the crabs legs will need to be cooked on a medium heat. Whilst the barbecue is heating up in a bowl mix together the olive oil and butter and then brush this over the crab legs.

2. Now place the crab legs on the grill, which you may want to lightly oil as well and close the lid on your barbecue. Now let the legs cook on the barbecue for between 4 and 5

minutes making sure that halfway through you turn them over.

3. Once the crabs legs are cooked remove from the barbecue and serve them with some fresh crusty bread along with a cocktail or garlic butter sauce. To make the garlic butter sauce in a sauce pan place 50grams of melted butter with 1 tablespoon of freshly chopped garlic and heat gently. Doing this will then allow the flavor of the garlic to become infused in the butter.

Recipe 2 – Spicy Shrimp Skewers

This is the perfect recipe to serve at any barbecue in the summer. The perfect accompaniment to this dish is seasoned rice along with frozen margaritas.

Ingredients

900grams Large Shrimps (Peeled and Deveined)
80ml Fresh Lime Juice
80ml Honey
1 Teaspoon Soy Sauce
1 Teaspoon Vegetable Oil
2 Tablespoons Jamaican Jerk Seasoning
3 Dashes Hot Pepper Sauce
Salt and Freshly Ground Black Pepper to Taste

12 Wooden Skewers That Have Been Soaked In Water For 1 Hour

Instructions

1. In a bowl combine together the lime juice, honey, soy sauce and oil. Then to this add the Jamaican jerk seasoning, hot pepper sauce, salt and pepper.

2. Now add to the sauce you have just made the shrimps make sure that you mix everything well together so that the shrimps are completely coated in the sauce. Cover the bowl and place in the refrigerator and leave there for one hour to allow the shrimps to marinate in the sauce. This is the time when the skewers should have been placed in the water to soak.

3. About 30 minutes before the shrimps are due to come out the refrigerator you should now get your barbecue going. The shrimps will need to be cooked on a medium to high heat so place the grill of the barbecue about 4 to 6 inches above the heat source.

4. After removing the shrimps from the refrigerator now remove the skewers from the water, then pat them dry before then spraying or brushing with some non stick cooking spray or oil. Now thread on to each skewer the shrimps until all 12 skewers have been used and place on the grill and cook each kebab for 5 minutes on each side or until the shrimps have turned pink in color.

Once the shrimps are cooked place on clean plates and serve with the seasoned rice and frozen margaritas

Recipe 3 – Grilled Oysters

It is important that you make sure that you clean the oysters very well. However you may find that they have already been cleaned well by your fishmonger and so will only need a light scrubbing and rinsing. Whilst you are cleaning the oysters make sure that they are tightly closed. If they aren't or you find that they are easy to open through them away as these aren't fresh or healthy. After cleaning them keep them cold by placing them in a bowl with a bag ice on top.

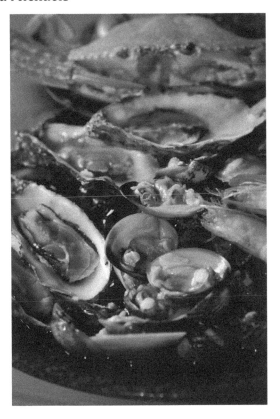

Ingredients

12 to 18 Oysters For Each Person
Melted Butter
Hot Sauce
Worcestershire Sauce

Instructions

1. Once the barbecue has heated up place the oysters on to the grill on a medium to high heat. If you want to prevent any flare ups

whilst the oysters are cooking as juices drip out of them then cover the grill with some aluminum foil first.

2. After placing the oysters on the grill close the lid of the barbecue and let them cook. It is important that you keep a close eye on the oysters as they are cooking. So check them every 3 to 4 minutes. Once you notice the shells starting to open then remove them from the grill.

3. After removing the oysters from the grill open the shells and then loosen the meat and place on a plate so your guests can then help themselves. Beside the plate of oysters put some bowls with the melted butter, hot sauce and Worcestershire sauce in them and which the guests can then spoon on top of the oysters if they wish. Then simply pop in the mouth and enjoy.

Recipe 4 – Thai Spiced Prawns

If you are looking for a barbecued prawn recipe that comes with a little kick then this is the one for you.

Ingredients

450grams Medium Size Prawns (Peeled and Deveined)
3 Tablespoons Fresh Lemon Juice
1 Tablespoon Soy Sauce
1 Tablespoon Dijon Mustard
2 Garlic Cloves Minced
1 Tablespoon Brown Sugar
2 Teaspoons Curry Paste

Instructions

1. In either a resealable plastic bag or a shallow baking dish mix together the lemon juice, soy sauce, mustard, garlic, sugar and curry paste. Then add the prawns and mix all these ingredients together thoroughly. Now seal up the bag or cover the dish with some cling film and place in the refrigerator to marinate for 1 hour.

2. Next heat up the barbecue and place the grill down low as you will be cooking these prawns on a high heat. Once the barbecue is ready lightly oil the grill and place the prawns that have been threaded onto skewers and cook on each side for 3 minutes each. If you want to make turning them over easier place the kebabs inside a fish basket. You will know when the prawns are ready, as they will turn a pink opaque color.

3. As for the remaining sauce, which you marinated the prawns in initially, transfer this to a small saucepan and heat up until it starts to boil. Allow it to boil for a few minutes before then transferring to a bowl which your guests can then dip the kebabs in and which you have also used to baste the prawns in whilst cooking.

Recipe 5 – Garlic Grilled Shrimps

You can serve these shrimps either with pasta or salad or as fajitas to your guests.

Ingredients

450grams Large Size Shrimps (Peeled and Deveined)
4 Garlic Cloves
Salt to Taste
30ml Olive Oil
¼ Teaspoon Freshly Ground Black Pepper to Taste

Instructions

1. Start the barbecue up and lightly oil the grill.

2. Now take the four garlic cloves and chop them up then sprinkle with some salt and using the back of a large knife smash the garlic up until it forms a paste. Then place the garlic with some olive oil in a frying pan (skillet) and cook over a medium to low heat until the garlic starts to turn brown. This should take around 5 minutes then once the garlic has turned brown remove from heat.

3. Next you take the shrimps and thread them onto wooden skewers and sprinkle over them some salt and pepper to season. Then brush one side of the shrimps with the garlic and olive oil mixture you made earlier and place this side down on to the barbecue.

4. Cook the shrimps until they start to turn pink in color and they begin to curl. This should take around 4 minutes and then turn them over. But before placing back down on the barbecue brush with more of the garlic oil and then cook for a further 4 minutes until the flesh has turned opaque and the shrimps are pink all over.

Recipe 6 – Bacon Wrapped Shrimps

Can either be served as an appetiser to your guests as they arrive or as a starter.

Ingredients

16 Large Shrimps (Peeled and Deveined)
8 Slices of Bacon
Barbecue Seasoning to Taste

Instructions

1. Preheat the barbecue and place the grill about 4 to 6 inches above the heat.

2. Take each shrimp and wrap them in half of each slice of bacon and then secure with a toothpick or thread two of them on to a wooden skewer that has been soaking in water for 30 minutes.

3. Now sprinkle some of the seasoning over them and then place each one on to the lightly oiled barbecue grill and cook for around 10 to 15 minutes. It is important that you turn the shrimps over frequently to prevent the bacon from burning and also to ensure that the

shrimps are cooked through evenly. Once cooked place on a clean plate and allow your guests to help themselves.

Recipe 7 – Scallops With A Herb & Pecan Crust

The crust that you coat the scallops with adds a very fresh accent to this delicious tasting seafood.

Ingredients

450grams Scallops (About 12 to 15 Scallops)
64grams Toasted Pecan Pieces
43grams Fresh Oregano Leaves
32grams Fresh Thyme Leaves
3 Garlic Cloves Chopped
2 Teaspoons Chicken Flavored Bouillon Granules
1 Teaspoon Freshly Shredded Lemon Peel
¼ Teaspoon Freshly Ground Black Pepper
3 Tablespoons Olive Oil

Instructions

1. In a food processor place the pecan pieces, oregano, thyme, garlic, bouillon granules, lemon peel and black pepper. Turn machine on until they form a paste then very slowly and gradually add the olive oil.

2. Once you have formed a paste now rub it onto the scallops and then thread three of each on to a skewer. If you are using wooden ones remember to soak in water for at least 30 minutes to prevent them from burning when on the barbecue.

3. Once the scallops are ready on the skewers place on the preheated barbecue over a medium heat so set the grill about 6 inches above the heat source and cook them for between 5 and 8 minutes. The best way of knowing when the scallops are ready to serve is to see if they have turned opaque in color.

4. As soon as the scallops are cooked serve to your guests on clean plates with some crusty bread and a crisp green salad that has been drizzled with lemon juice and olive oil

Recipe 8 – Grilled Oysters With Fennel Butter

This particular recipe cannot only be served as a main dish to your guests but as an accompaniment to others.

Ingredients

24 Fresh Live Unopened Medium Size Oysters
1 Teaspoon Grounded Fennel Seed
226grams Softened Butter
1 Tablespoon Minced Shallots
1 Tablespoon Chopped Fennel Greens
1 Teaspoon Freshly Ground Black Pepper
½ Teaspoon Salt

Instructions

1. Get the barbecue going so and place the grill down low as possible as you will be cooking the oysters on a very high heat.

2. In a bowl mix together the butter, fennel seeds, shallots, fennel greens, pepper and salt. Then put to one side for use later. If you want place in the refrigerator to keep the butter from

melting completely and remove about 10 minutes before needed.

3. Place the oysters on the grill of the barbecue and close the lid and leave it closed for between 3 and 5 minutes or until you start to hear them hiss or they start to open.

4. Take an oyster knife and pry each one of the oysters open at the hinge and loosen the oyster inside. Discard the flat part of the shell and then top each of the open oysters with ½ teaspoon of the butter you made earlier and then return them back to the barbecue once more. Then cook them once more until the butter has melted and is hot.

Recipe 9 – Grilled Crab

Most people don't think that cooking things such as crabs on a barbecue is a good idea. But it is because the direct heat and flavor help to make this one of the best ways of cooking most types of shellfish today.

Ingredients

2 Large Live Crabs
60ml White Wine Vinegar
2 ½ Teaspoons Sugar
2 Tablespoons Olive Oil
1 Tablespoon Freshly Minced Ginger
1 Jalapeno Chilli Seeds Removed Then Minced
1 Tablespoon Minced Cilantro
1 Medium Tomato Chopped

Instructions

1. In a bowl mix together the chopped tomato, vinegar, oil, ginger, chilli, garlic and cilantro. Then place to one side for use later.

2. Now into a large pot of boiling water place the crabs one at the time head first. Reduce the

heat and allow the crabs to sit in simmering water for 5 minutes before then removing. If however you find the thought of cooking live crabs a little too much then you can use frozen ones instead. Of course you need to allow them sufficient time to thaw out before you can start cooking with them.

3.   After removing the crabs from the water turn over and pull the triangular tab from the belly and lift of the shell. Remove the entrails and gills from the crab before then washing and draining. Now place on the barbecue that you have preheated and close the lid. But before closing the lid brush with the mixture you made earlier and do this regularly throughout the time the crabs are grilling on the barbecue.

4. About halfway through the cooking time (around about 5minutes) you need to turn the crabs over and repeat the same process again for a further 5 minutes or until the meat in the legs of the crabs has turned opaque.

5. Now place the crabs on to a plate to serve them but before you do serve spoon over any remaining sauce you have that you used to baste the crabs in when cooking. If you wish

you can put the meat back in the shells before serving.

Recipe 10 – Sesame Scallops

This marinade helps to enhance the flavor of the scallops even further. Best served either on a bed of noodles, rice or with some grilled vegetables.

Ingredients

900grams Fresh Sea Scallops
60ml Vegetable Oil
60ml Distilled White Vinegar
2 Tablespoons Hoisin Sauce
2 Tablespoons Soy Sauce
2 Tablespoons Dry Sherry
1 Tablespoon Freshly Minced Ginger
1 Teaspoon Sesame Oil
1 Garlic Clove Minced
1 Green Onion Minced
Sesame Seeds

Instructions

1. First off wash and then pat dry with some paper towels the scallops.

2. Now into a bowl mix together the oil, vinegar, hoisin and soy sauce, dry sherry,

ginger, sesame oil, garlic and onion. Then pour this mixture into a resealable bag and then add to these the scallops. Turn the bag over several times to ensure that all the scallops are covered in the marinade and place in the refrigerator overnight.

3. Whilst the barbecue is heating up you can now remove the scallops from the refrigerator and thread them on to skewers ready for cooking. Once placed on the skewers then sprinkle over some of the sesame seeds and cook over a medium heat (so place the grill about 4 to 6 inches above the heat source) and cook for 6 to 8 minutes. You will know the scallops are ready to eat when they have turned opaque.

Recipe 11 – Margarita Shrimps

If you wish you can marinate the shrimps in this sauce for up to 3 hours. Plus you can increase or reduce the amount of red pepper included in this dish dependent on how hot you like your food to be.

Ingredients

450grams Shrimps (Peeled and Deveined)
2 Garlic Cloves Minced
2 Tablespoons Fresh Lime Juice
3 Tablespoons Olive Oil
2 Teaspoons Tequila
3 Tablespoons Freshly Chopped Cilantro
¼ Teaspoon Ground Red Pepper
¼ Teaspoon Salt

Instructions

1. In a bowl place the lime juice, olive oil, tequila, garlic, cilantro, pepper and salt and combine well together before then adding the shrimps. Toss the mixture about lightly to ensure that the shrimps are covered in the sauce then cover the bowl and place in the

refrigerator for between 30 minutes and 3 hours to marinate.

2. Turn on or light the barbecue about 30 minutes prior to when you want to start cooking the shrimps. You need to place the grill down low in the barbecue, as you will be cooking these on a high heat for a very short space of time.

3. Whilst the barbecue is heating up take the shrimps out of the fridge and thread them on to either metal or wooden skewers. Put about 3 or 4 on each skewer and place to one side. If there is any marinade left over in the bowl discard this.

4. Before you place the shrimps on to the barbecue grill lightly oil it first to prevent the shrimps from sticking to it. Now cook the shrimps for between 2 and 3 minutes on each side or until they have turned pink. Then serve.

Recipe 12 – Baja Style Grilled Rock Lobster Tails

This very simple citrus sauce complements the richness of the lobster tails very well. Best served with warm tortillas and lightly grilled green onions. To cut the tails in half you should use either kitchen shears or a cleaver. If you want to give this dish a more authentic Mexican flavor then douse the tails in a hot Mexican sauce like Cholula.

Ingredients
6 x 226gram Rock Or Spiny Lobster Tails
12 Green Onions

Sauce

1 Tablespoon Grated Orange Rind
2 Tablespoons Freshly Squeezed Orange Juice
1 Tablespoon Freshly Squeezed Lemon Juice
1 Tablespoon Olive Oil
½ Teaspoon Dried Oregano
¼ Teaspoon Salt
Dash of Hot Sauce (Such as Cholula)
1 Garlic Clove Minced
2 Tablespoons Melted Butter

Instructions

1. Get the barbecue going so it is ready in time for cooking to begin.

2. Now you need to start preparing the lobster. To do this cut each lobster tail in half lengthwise and then coat each one along with the onions with some cooking spray.

3. Next place the tails on to the grill of the barbecue cut side facing downwards and after you have oiled the grill lightly. Grill the tails for 3 minutes and then turn them over. Now grill them for a further five minutes.

4. About 2 minutes after turning over the tails now place the green onions on the grill to

cook. These will require about 3 minutes and should be turned over at least once during this cooking time. Remove from barbecue once they have become tender.

5. To make the sauce which you will serve with the lobster tails in to a bowl place the orange rind, orange juice, lime juice, olive oil, oregano, salt, hot sauce and garlic and whisk well. Then very gradually add to this mixture the melted butter making sure that you whisk the ingredients continuously then drizzle it over the cut side of the tails.

6. Transfer to a clean plate and serve alongside them some warm tortillas and some lime wedges.

Recipe 13 – Grilled Prawns With Spicy Peanut Lime Vinaigrette

Not only does this Thai inspired sauce go very well with prawns but you may also want to try it with chicken, lamb or pork.

Ingredients

900grams (16-20) Extra Large Shrimps (Peeled and Deveined But Tails Left On)
32grams Minced Lemon Grass (White Part Only)
32grams Fresh Minced Ginger Root
2 Tablespoons Minced Garlic
¼ Tablespoon Freshly Chopped Cilantro
1 Thai or Serrano Chilli Minced
180ml Peanut or Canola Oil

Vinaigrette

60ml Lime Juice
60ml Rice Wine Vinegar
120ml Japanese Sweet Wine (Mirin)
2 Tablespoons Dark Soy Sauce
2 Tablespoons Cold Water
3 Tablespoons Grated Lime Zest
1 Tablespoon Freshly Minced Ginger Root

2 Teaspoons Fish Sauce
2 Fresh Thai or Serrano Chilli's (Seeds Removed)
2 Teaspoons Minced Garlic
113grams Unsalted Smooth Peanut Butter
30ml Peanut Oil
2 Tablespoons Freshly Chopped Mint
1 Tablespoon Freshly Chopped Cilantro
57grams Chopped Unsalted Roasted Peanuts
Salt to Taste

Instructions

1. In a bowl (large) combine together the ginger, lemon grass, garlic, cilantro, chilli and oil. Then add the shrimps and let them marinate in the sauce made for 20 to 30 minutes at room temperature.

2. Whilst the shrimps are marinating in the sauce you can now start heating up the barbecue placing the grill about 6 inches above the heat source. This will then enable you to cook the shrimps that you will thread on to skewers on a medium to high heat.

3. Now into a food processor place the lime juice, rice vinegar, mirin, soy sauce and water and blend. Then add to this the lime zest,

ginger, fish sauce, chillis, garlic and peanut butter and process until the mixture becomes smooth. Whilst these ingredients are combining together slowly pour in the peanut oil until the mixture looks smooth and creamy.

Pour this mixture into a bowl and then stir into it the mint, cilantro and chopped peanuts. Add some salt if needed.

4. To cook the shrimps remove them from the marinade, shaking off any excess and thread them on to skewers then cook them on either side for about 2 minutes or until they have turned pink and firm. Once cooked serve on a plate immediately with the sauce beside them.

Recipe 14 – Scallops & Cherry Tomato Kebabs

The applying of fresh lemon juice and Dijon mustard to these scallops and tomato kebabs helps to give them a much spicier and tarter flavor.

Ingredients

16 Large Sea Scallops
24 Cherry Tomatoes
1 Lemon
2 Tablespoons Olive Oil
2 Tablespoons Dijon Mustard
1/8 Teaspoon Salt

Instructions

1. Start preparing the barbecue for cooking this dish on a medium heat. This means putting the grill of the barbecue about 6 inches above the main heat source. Also place the wooden skewers in some water.

2. Whilst the barbecue is heating up you can now prepare the sauce for the kebabs. In a bowl place 1 tablespoon of lemon juice along

with ½ teaspoon of its peel. To this then add the olive oil, Dijon mustard and salt and mix well together. Then put to one side ready for use later.

3. Now on to each of the wooden skewers you need to thread 3 tomatoes and 2 scallops alternately. You should start and finish with the tomatoes.

4. Next brush the kebabs you have just made with some of the sauce you made earlier and place on the barbecue to cook. Each kebab will need to cook for between 7 and 9 minutes and should be turned over several times. After this time has elapsed brush the kebabs with the remainder of the sauce and then cook for another 5 minutes or more remembering to turn them over frequently. The kebabs will be ready to consume when the scallops have turned opaque right through.

5. Once the kebabs are cooked served to your guests immediately with a little green salad and some crusty bread.

Recipe 15 – Grilled Lobster With Lime Bay Butter

This is quite an easy dish to do. However before the lobsters are placed on the barbecue they need to be parboiled first.

Ingredients

3 x 680grams Fresh Lobsters
113grams Butter
60ml Fresh Lime Juice
½ Teaspoon Crushed Bay Leaf
¼ Teaspoon Freshly Ground Black Pepper
¼ Teaspoon Salt

Instructions

1. To parboil the lobsters you need to bring around 3 inches of water to boil in an 8 quart saucepan. Once the water begins boiling add the lobsters, then cover the pan and cook for 10 minutes. Once the 10 minutes has elapsed remove the lobsters from the pan and leave them to one side to cool.

2. Whilst the barbecue is heating up in another saucepan place the butter, lime juice, bay leaf,

salt and pepper and cook for 10 minutes over a low heat. Then put to one side to use later on.

3. By now the lobsters should have cooled down sufficiently to enable you to cut them in half lengthwise and brush them with the butter mixture you have just made.

4. After brushing the cut side of the lobster with the butter mixture you place them cut side down onto the grill of the barbecue which you have placed about 4 inches above the heat source and cook them for 5 minutes.

5. Now turn the lobsters over carefully brushing them with some more of the butter mixture and continuing cooking them on the barbecue until the meat is cooked through. This should take about another 5 minutes.

6. As soon as the meat is cooked through remove the lobsters from the barbecue place on a clean plate and garnish them with lime wedges and bay leaves if you want. Each of your guests should be given ½ lobster each

Recipe 16 – Grilled Prawns & Garlic Chilli Sauce

The sauce you use with this particular recipe helps to enhance the sweetness of the prawns even further. Don't be surprised if you guests won't to know the secret to this great tasting dish.

Ingredients

450grams Jumbo Size Prawns (Devein Them)
2 Tablespoons Cooking Oil
2 Tablespoons Minced Garlic
2 Tablespoons Thinly Sliced Lemon Grass
5 Fresh Thai Chilli's Thinly Sliced
1 Shallot Thinly Sliced
2 Kaffir Lime Leaves
1 Tablespoon Fish Sauce
Juice Of 1 Lime
1 Tablespoon Thai Roasted Chilli Paste
1 Tablespoon Torn Fresh Mint Leaves

Instructions

1. Turn on or light your barbecue ready for cooking the prawns on. Placing the grill which has been lightly oiled about 6 inches above the

heat sauce allowing you to cook the prawns on a medium heat.

2. Once the barbecue is heated up now place the prawns on to the grill and cook until the outside starts to turn pink and the meat inside not longer looks transparent. They will need to cook for between 5 and 10 minutes and should be turned over frequently. Whilst they are cooking you should now be making the sauce, which the prawns can then be dipped into.

3. To make the sauce heat some oil over a medium heat in a skillet and to this then add the garlic until it turns brown, which should take around 7 to 10 minutes. Now remove from the heat and to the oil and garlic add the lemon grass, chillis, shallot, lime leaves, fish sauce, lime juice and chilli paste. Toss to combine all these ingredients together then spoon some of them over the prawns, which you have removed from the barbecue and placed on a serving dish and the rest you pour into a bowl. Garnish with the freshly torn mint leaves.

Recipe 17 – Grilled New England Seafood

If you are looking for a recipe that doesn't take a great deal to prepare and won't leave you with too much mess afterwards this is one you should consider trying.

Ingredients

450grams Skinless Cod Fillet (Cut Into Four Equal Pieces)
225grams Frozen Uncooked Prawns (Peeled and Deveined and Thawed)
225grams Red New Potatoes (Skins Scrubbed then Thinly Sliced)
2 Ears of Corn Quartered
2 Tablespoons Butter (Room Temperature)
2 Tablespoons Finely Chopped Fresh Dill
1 Small Garlic Clove Minced
Coarse Salt and Freshly Ground Black Pepper To Taste
1 Lemon Thinly Sliced

Instructions

1. Start by getting your barbecue going and place the grill 6 inches above the heat source

to allow the packets you are about to make to cook on a medium heat.

2. Whilst the barbecue is heating up in a bowl mix together the butter, dill, garlic, salt and pepper and place to one side for now.

3. Take four squares of aluminum foil measuring 14 inches square each. On to each of these four pieces of foil first place the thinly sliced potatoes before then placing on top of them a piece of the cod.

Next lay on some of the prawns and alongside the potatoes; cod and prawns place two pieces of the corn. Season each parcel with salt and pepper before adding a spoonful of the butter mixture on top. Then place on top of these two slices of the lemon.

4. Now bring up the sides of the foil and crimp the edges to seal the ingredients inside them tightly. Place each parcel on to the grill making sure that the potato is on the bottom and cook for about 12 to 14 minutes or until the fish is just cooked through and the potatoes are tender. You should make sure that you rotate not flip the parcels occasionally as this

will help to ensure that everything inside is cooked properly.

5. Once the cooking time has passed remove the parcels from the heat and slit open the top of each one and transfer the contents to plates. If you want garnish the food with some more dill sprigs and serve some warm crusty rolls with them.

Recipe 18 – Honey Grilled Shrimps

Adding onions, peppers and mushrooms to this dish really helps to bring out even more of the beautiful flavors of the shrimps. You may also want to consider marinating the vegetables in the sauce along with the shrimps.

Ingredients

450grams Large Shrimps (Peeled and Deveined but with Tails still attached)
½ Teaspoon Garlic Powder
¼ Tablespoon Freshly Ground Black Pepper
80ml Worcestershire Sauce
2 Tablespoons Dry White Wine
2 Tablespoons Italian Style Salad Dressing

Honey Sauce

60ml Honey
57grams Melted Butter
2 Tablespoons Worcestershire Sauce

Instructions

1. Into a large bowl mix together the garlic powder, black pepper, Worcestershire sauce,

dry white wine and the salad dressing. Then add the shrimp and toss them to coat them evenly in the marinade. Now cover the bowl over and place in the refrigerator to let the shrimp marinate in the sauce for 1 hour.

2. Start the barbecue up and place the grill, which needs to be lightly, oiled about 4 inches above the heat source to allow the shrimps to cook on a high heat. Remove the shrimps from the marinade and thread onto skewers. Pierce one through the head then the next one through the tail. Any marinade left over can now be discarded. Then set the shrimps to one side for a moment whilst you make the honey sauce.

3. To make the honey sauce in a small bowl mix together the honey melted butter and the other 2 tablespoons of Worcestershire sauce. This is what you will be basting the shrimps in as they cook.

4. Take the shrimps and place on the lightly oiled grill and cook for 2 to 3 minutes on each side, making sure you baste them occasionally with the honey sauce you have just made. You will know when the shrimps are ready to serve because the flesh will have turned opaque

throughout. Serve to your guests immediately once cooked.

Recipe 19 – Scallops Wrapped In Prosciutto

These will make a great starter to any barbecue and because they contain so few ingredients not only are they easy to prepare but also easy to cook.

Ingredients

900grams (40) Medium Sized Scallops
450grams Paper Thin Slices Prosciutto
2 Lemons Halved
Freshly Ground Black Pepper
Extra Virgin Olive Oil (For Drizzling)

Instructions

1. Turn your gas barbecue on to high and allow to heat up whilst you are preparing the scallops for cooking. If you are using a charcoal barbecue you will know when it is hot enough when you can only hold your hand over it about 5 inches above the grill for 2 seconds.

2. Take one slice of the prosciutto and cut in half lengthwise then fold in half and wrap it

around the sides of a scallop. You need to make sure that the ends of the prosciutto overlap and then thread it on to a skewer. Do the same for the other pieces of prosciutto and the scallops.

3. Next take the olive oil and drizzle it lightly over the scallops and then squeeze some lemon juice over them. Then season with the freshly ground black pepper. Then place on the barbecue to cook. Cook on each side for about 3 minutes or until you see the flesh of the scallops has turned opaque.

Remove from barbecue place on a clean plate with some lemon wedges and serve to your guests.

Recipe 20 – Maple Orange Shrimp & Scallop Kebabs

Your guests will love the combination of the scallops and shrimps with the sweet citrus glaze. Make a wonderful entrée or starter to your barbecue. If you intend to serve as an entrée then place just one scallop and shrimp onto each skewer. If you intend to serve them as main course then serve with either steamed rice or seasonal vegetables or with a mixed green salad and light vinaigrette.

Ingredients

12 Jumbo Shrimps (Peeled and Deveined)
12 Large Sea Scallops
3 Tablespoons Vegetable Oil
½ Teaspoon Salt
½ Teaspoon Freshly Ground Black Pepper
120ml Tomato Ketchup
60ml Orange Juice
60ml Maple Syrup
1 Tablespoon Worcestershire Sauce
1 Tablespoon Apple Cider Vinegar
½ Teaspoon Paprika
3 Garlic Cloves Minced

Instructions

1. Onto a skewer thread 3 scallops and 3 shrimps alternately. Then brush with the vegetable before seasoning with the salt and pepper. Then place to one side for cooking later.

2. In a bowl put the ketchup, orange juice, maple syrup, Worcestershire sauce, apple cider vinegar, paprika and garlic and combine well together. This you will then be used for basting the scallops and shrimps as they cook on the barbecue. So set to onside until you start cooking.

3. Whilst you are doing the various tasks above you should be getting your barbecue started with the grill be set about 4 to 6 inches above the heat source so the food can cook on a medium to high heat.

4. As soon as your barbecue is ready lightly oil the grill and then place the shrimp and scallop kebabs on it. But just before you do brush the kebabs all over with the maple orange sauce and then baste them with it regularly. Each side of these kebabs should be allowed to cook for 2 to 3 minutes or until the flesh of the scallops and shrimps have turned opaque.

Recipe 21 – Ginger Shrimp With Charred Tomato Relish

Green tomatoes quite simply are ones that haven't ripened yet. Not only do they have slightly sour taste to them but also contain less sugar. By charring them you will find that they are a lot easier to peel because they have become softer.

Ingredients

20 Extra Large Shrimps (Peeled, Deveined but Tails Left On)
2 Garlic Cloves Minced
1 ½ Tablespoons Grated Peeled Ginger
3 Tablespoons Vegetable Oil
4 Ripe Plum Tomatoes (Cut In Half Lengthwise)
2 Medium Green Tomatoes (Cut In Half Lengthwise)
Coarse Salt
Freshly Ground Black Pepper
2 Tablespoons Fresh Lime Juice
1 Tablespoon Freshly Minced Jalapeno Chilli (With Seeds)
1 Teaspoon Sugar
1 Tablespoon Freshly Chopped Cilantro

1 Tablespoon Freshly Chopped Basil

Instructions

1. In to a bowl mix together the garlic and ginger. Now take half of this and transfer to another bowl and add to these 2 tablespoons of the oil before then adding the shrimps and tossing them in the mixture to make sure that they are evenly coated in it. Now cover this bowl over and place in the refrigerator for 30 minutes to allow the shrimps to marinate. As for the rest of the ginger and garlic mixture this should be covered and placed in the refrigerator as well.

2. Now heat up the barbecue and whilst this is happening into another bowl put the tomatoes and toss them in the last tablespoon of oil along with some salt and pepper to season. Now grill the tomatoes on the barbecue the cut sides facing upwards until the skins become charred and the flesh inside becomes tender.

The plum tomatoes will take around 4 to 6 minutes to cook and the green tomatoes will take about 8 to 10 minutes to cook. If the green tomatoes are especially hard they may need a little longer than 10 minutes.

Also be careful when cooking the tomatoes as both the juices from them and the oil in which they are coated may cause flare ups to occur.

3. Once the skins have become charred on the tomatoes and the flesh soft remove from heat and set to one side to allow them to cool down a little. As soon as they have cooled down enough peel away and discard the skins and seeds then finely chop them up and add to the garlic and ginger mixture from earlier. Also add to this mixture the lime juice, jalapeno chilli, sugar cilantro and basil then well combined together pour into a serving dish and set to one side for later.

4. Remove shrimps from refrigerator and just before placing on to the barbecue thread one shrimp on to a skewer through both the top and tail and sprinkle with some salt and pepper. Place on the barbecue and cook for about 2 minutes on each side or until the flesh has turned opaque throughout.

Once cooked place the skewers on to a clean plate along with the bowl of tomato relish you made earlier.

Recipe 22 – Shrimp & Broccoli Packets

If you want to serve your guests with a flavorsome but fuss free meal then this one should be considered.

Ingredients

225grams Medium Size Shrimps (Peeled and Deveined)
175grams Instant Rice
2 Teaspoons Seafood Seasoning
2 Garlic Cloves Minced
220grams Broccoli Florets
2 Tablespoons Butter (Cut Into Pieces)
8 Ice Cubes
120ml Water

Instructions

1. Preheat the barbecue and place the grill about 4 to 6 inches above the heat source so you can cook these parcels on a medium to high heat.

2. Whilst the barbecue is heating up place half the shrimps on a piece of aluminum foil with the non stick (dull) side facing up towards the

food. Then around this arrange half the rice and sprinkle it and the shrimps with some of the seafood seasoning before then topping off the shrimps with half the minced garlic. Then place half the broccoli on top of the shrimp and sprinkle with garlic and butter. Do the same for the other parcel and then top each one off with 4 ice cubes.

3. Now bring the sides of the aluminum foil up and double fold over the top and at one end. At the end, which is still open, pour in half the water and then fold this end over so that the ingredients are now sealed inside. Make sure that you use a large enough piece of foil to allow room for heat and steam to circulate inside.

4. Once the parcels are ready place on the barbecue and let them cook for 9 to 13 minutes. It is important that you close the lid whilst the parcels are cooking to ensure that things cook evenly.

5. After removing from the grill snip open the parcels and stir the rice before you then serve as they are to your guests. It is also a good idea to squeeze some fresh lemon juice over the shrimps, rice and broccoli just before serving.

Recipe 23 – Tangy Shrimp & Scallops

After cooking serve these kebabs with pasta, green salad and some garlic bread.

Ingredients

28 Large Shrimps (Peeled & Deveined)
28 Large Sea Scallops
113grams Butter or Margarine
7 Tablespoons Lemon Juice (Fresh Would Be Ideal)
5 Tablespoons Worcestershire Sauce
1 Teaspoon Garlic Powder
1 Teaspoon Paprika

Instructions

1. In a large resealable bag place the scallops and shrimps.

2. Now into a bowl (that can be used safely in a microwave) place the butter or margarine, the lemon juice, Worcestershire sauce, garlic powder and paprika. Cook on 50% power for about 1 to 1 ½ minutes or until the butter/margarine is melted then stir to ensure that all these ingredients are blended together.

3. Once the sauce is made set aside about a third of it as this you will then use to baste the shrimps and scallops in whilst they are cooking. As for the rest of the sauce this must be poured over the scallops and shrimps in the bag. Now seal the bag and turn it over several times to ensure that every scallop and shrimp is coated in the sauce and place in the refrigerator for one hour. Whilst in the refrigerator make sure that you turn the back over occasionally.

3. Whilst the barbecue is heating up you can now prepare the kebabs. Take some wooden skewers that have been soaking in water and thread alternately on to them the scallops and shrimps.

4. Once all the kebabs are made place them on the preheated barbecue and cook them on a medium to hot heat for 6 minutes turning once during this time. Both before and during this cooking time baste them occasionally with the sauce you set to one side earlier. Then cook them for a further 8 to 10 minutes or longer until the shrimps have turned pink and the scallops opaque.

Recipe 24 – Barbecued Oysters Served With Hogwash

Looking for something special to serve at your next barbecue to your guests then why not give this recipe a go.

Ingredients

48 Oysters (Scrubbed)

Hogwash

120ml Natural Rice Vinegar
120ml Seasoned Rice Vinegar
2 Finely Chopped Shallots
3 Tablespoons Freshly Squeezed (Strained) Lime Juice
1 Small Jalapeno Chilli (Seeded and Finely Chopped)
Fresh Roughly Chopped Cilantro

Instructions

1. Heat up the barbecue until it is very hot then place the unopened fresh oysters on to the lightly oiled grill and close the lid. After about 3 minutes check to see if the oysters are open.

2. If the oysters are open then detach the oysters from the top shell using an oyster knife. Then loosen the top shells and discard these. Then you simply need to place a spoonful of the Hogwash sauce you have made over each one before serving them.

3. In order to make the Hogwash place the seasoned and natural rice vinegar into a bowl with the shallots, lime juice, jalapeno chilli and cilantro and mix well together. You should make this before you actually begin cooking the oysters, as it needs to go into the refrigerator for at least an hour.

Recipe 25 – Scallops, Orange & Cucumber Kebabs

Yet another very simple recipe you may want to try but is one that really helps to enhance the amazing flavors of the scallops. It is important that you use the freshest scallops possible.

Ingredients

450grams Large Scallops
8 Very Thin Slices Peeled Fresh Ginger
2 Tablespoons Honey
120ml Fresh Orange Juice
½ Navel Orange Cut Into Wedges
½ Cucumber Cut In Half Lengthways Then Cut Into ½ Inch Slices
Coarse Salt
Freshly Ground Black Pepper

Instructions

1. Start by getting the barbecue heated up. You will need to place the lightly oiled grill about 6 inches above the heat source as you want to

cook these kebabs on a medium heat to ensure that nothing burns.

2. Whilst the barbecue is heating up in a small bowl mix together the honey and orange juice and set to one side for later.

3. Next take four skewers (wooden ones will do but you can use metal ones if you want). On to these thread an orange wedge followed by a slice of ginger, cucumber and scallop until each skewer is full. Also make sure that you end with another wedge of orange on the kebabs.

4. Now season each kebab with salt and pepper before then brushing with the orange and honey sauce made earlier. Place each kebab on to the grill of the barbecue and cook for between 4 and 6 minutes or until the scallop flesh has turned opaque. Make sure that you turn the kebabs frequently and baste regularly with the sauce.

Once the kebabs are cooked serve with some rice or a crisp green salad.

Recipe 26 – Prawns With Pistou

If you wish rather than using prawns you can use large shrimps instead.

Ingredients

12 Prawns (Shelled and Deveined But With Heads Left On)
27.5grams Whole Raw Almonds
128grams Loose Packed Fresh Flat Leaf Parsley
12 Anchovy Fillets (Rinsed)
2 Garlic Cloves (Peeled)
60ml Extra Virgin Olive Oil
2 Tablespoons Extra Virgin Olive Oil
Zest of 1 Lemon
Coarse Salt
Freshly Ground Black Pepper

Instructions

1. Take the whole raw almonds and place in the oven on a baking tray for 10 minutes at 350 degrees Fahrenheit. Stir the almonds occasionally and remove from oven when golden brown and fragrant. Then allow to cool

down completely before coarsely chopping them.

2. Now take the coarsely chopped almonds and place them in food processor with the basil, parsley, anchovies and garlic and process until all have been combined together. Then to this paste add the oil very slowly in a steady stream and continue processing until a smooth paste is formed.

Now transfer this mixture to a large bowl and mix in the lemon zest, salt and pepper. Put around a ¼ of this mixture to one side, as this is what your guests will then dip the shrimps in after they are cooked.

3. Whilst you are preparing the Pistou you should be allowing the barbecue to heat up ready for cooking. Place the grill about 5 inches above the heat source, as you will want to cook the shrimps on a medium to high heat.

4. As soon as the barbecue is ready toss the shrimps in the rest of the Pistou and place them on the barbecue and cook for about 2 ½ minutes on each side. Plus before placing on the barbecue season with some salt and pepper. You should only turn the shrimps over

once during the cooking time and to make sure that they are cooked through the flesh should be firm and they should have turned pink.

5. As soon as the shrimps are cooked place onto a clean plate with some lemon wedges and the bowl of Pistou you put to one side earlier. Your guests can then dip the shrimps into this.

Recipe 27 – Black & White Pepper Shrimps

If you can use sustainable peppercorns for this particular recipe. You are going to find that this is a recipe that will prove a favorite with everyone.

Ingredients

450grams Jumbo Shrimps (Heads Still On But Peeled & Deveined)
1 Tablespoon Black Peppercorns
2 Teaspoons White Peppercorns
1 ½ Tablespoons Maldon Sea Salt
3 Tablespoons Safflower Oil

8 Sprigs Fresh Cilantro For Garnish

Instructions

1. In a shallow dish place 8 wooden skewers measuring 10 inches in cold water for at least 10 minutes.

2. Now start the barbecue up putting the grill about 6 inches above the heat source so that

the shrimps can cook on a medium to high heat.

3. Whilst the barbecue is heating up thread the shrimps on to the skewers starting with at the tail and threading through the body until it comes out of the head. Now put each one of these on to a baking tray for now.

4. In a mortar place the peppercorns and coarsely grind them together with a pestle. Then transfer these to a small bowl and mix into them the sea salt.

5. Just before you place the shrimps on the barbecue drizzle them with the oil (both sides) and then sprinkle with the peppercorn and salt mixture.

6. Now place the shrimps on the lightly oiled barbecue grill and cook until the prawns become a light pink color and slightly charred. This should take around 2 minutes to occur then turn the shrimps over and cook for about the same amount of time again.

7. To serve place the shrimps on a place and sprinkle with the sprigs of cilantro and a dipping sauce in a bowl.

Recipe 28 – Grilled Calamari

To avoid your calamari from becoming too chewy you need to either cook it really fast or really slow. When cooked serve it in a large bowl or as individual servings to your guests.

Ingredients

450grams Fresh Calamari (Cleaned, Rinsed & Well Dried)
60ml Extra Virgin Olive Oil
1 ½ Tablespoons Fresh Lemon Juice (About 1 Small Lemon)
1 Garlic Clove Thinly Sliced
2 Sprigs of Fresh Oregano or ½ Teaspoon Dried Oregano
½ Teaspoon Coarse Salt
Freshly Ground Black Pepper

Instructions

1. In a bowl place the olive oil; lemon juice and salt then stir until they combined together. Then into this mix the garlic and the whole sprigs or dried oregano.

2. Whilst you are making up this sauce you should be getting the barbecue heated up and place the grill down as low as possible in order to cook the calamari quick on a very high heat.

3. When the barbecue has heated up place the squid on the oiled grill and char each side of it for 1 minute. Now remove from the barbecue and slice all parts of the calamari including the tendrils cross wise into ¼ inch rings. Then add the calamari to the lemon sauce made earlier and then place on a serving plate. Just before you serve this dish to your guests make sure that you sprinkle over some freshly ground black pepper.

MORE 70 BEST EVER RECIPES EBOOKS REVEALED AT MY AUTHOR PAGE:-

CLICK HERE TO ACCESS THEM NOW